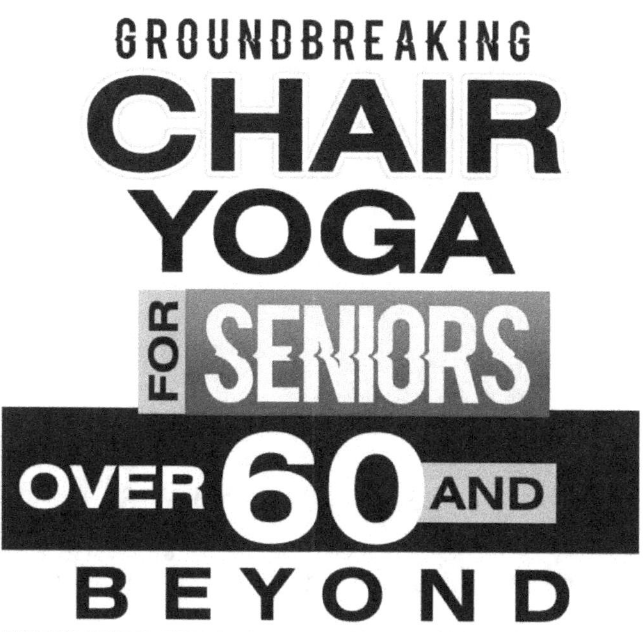

A Simple Exercise Challenge to Enhance Strength,
Flexibility, and Balance & Shed Pounds in Just
10 Minutes a Day, Including Tested Recipes

DR. JESSICA
REEVES

APPENDIX

QUICK REFERENCE MATERIALS

- RECIPE INDEX: QUICK ACCESS TO YOUR FAVORITE MEALS

- THE RECIPE FOR RECIPE ORGANIZATION

- WHY CREATE YOUR RECIPE BOOK TEMPLATE?

- INGREDIENTS FOR YOUR RECIPE BOOK

- INDEX OR TABLE OF CONTENTS

Introduction

CHAIR YOGA FOR SENIORS: A PATH TO HEALTH AND VITALITY FOR THE ELDERLY

Taking care of one's health and energy becomes an important priority at a later age. Welcome to the domain of "Yoga for Seniors in a Chair," a peaceful yet powerful practice meant to inspire older folks on their road to overall well-being. Come and experience chair yoga with us as we delve into its life-changing benefits for seniors, brought to you by Access Health Care Physicians, LLC.

Adopting a Lifestyle of Health and Vitality

1. Yoga for Elders: A Chair-Based Introduction

Step inside a sanctuary where every breath becomes a step towards healing and energy. Learn the basics of chair yoga for seniors and how it may help you feel better.

2. Access Health Care Physicians, LLC: Your Partner in Senior Wellness

Welcome to Access Health Care Physicians, LLC, your committed partner in achieving optimal health. Learn about their dedication to comprehensive elder care, combining chair yoga into a holistic approach to energy and well-being.

3. Chair Yoga for Seniors: The Core of Empowerment

Learn the many ways in which chair yoga may improve the mental, emotional, and physical well-being of seniors. It becomes a tool for self-care, resilience, and a revitalized sense of vigor.

4. Improved Flexibility and Mobility

Explore how chair yoga promotes flexibility and mobility, addressing typical issues experienced by seniors and encouraging a sense of freedom in movement.

5. Stress Reduction and Relaxation

Discover the stress-relieving advantages of chair yoga, as seniors embrace attentive breathing and gentle movements, creating a space for relaxation and mental calm.

6. Enhanced Balance and Stability

Delve into the ways chair yoga fosters better balance and stability, giving seniors the tools to manage daily life with confidence and enthusiasm.

7. Mindful Meditation for Mental Clarity

Engage in mindful meditation as part of chair yoga, building mental clarity, attention, and a positive mentality, leading to overall well-being.

8. Chair Yoga Nidra for Deep Relaxation

Explore Chair Yoga Nidra, a practice that goes beyond relaxation, allowing seniors to tap into deep sources of vitality, aiding both physical and mental restoration.

9. Seated Sun Salutation for Energy Boost

Experience the Seated Sun Salutation, a vigorous sequence that gives an energy boost, energizing the body and uplifting the spirit.

10. Chair Warrior III for Strength and Vitality

Adapt the Warrior III posture to the chair, inspiring elders with strength and vigor, providing a sense of success and perseverance.

11. Incorporating Chair Yoga into Daily Life

Learn practical methods to apply chair yoga into daily life, allowing seniors to weave the benefits smoothly into their routines for prolonged vitality.

12. Access Health Care Physicians, LLC Wellness Programs

Explore the specialized wellness programs offered by Access Health Care Physicians, LLC, combining chair yoga into a comprehensive approach for seniors to embrace energy and well-being.

Conclusion: A Journey to Vibrant Senior Living

As we continue our examination of Yoga for Seniors in a Chair, visualize a path where well-being and energy interweave. Access Health Care Physicians, LLC, invites seniors to embrace the transforming potential of chair yoga, opening a lively chapter in the golden years.

Frequently Asked Questions (FAQS)

1. Is chair yoga acceptable for elders with chronic health conditions?

Absolutely! Chair yoga may be tailored to fit varied health issues, giving a gentle and accessible type of exercise.

2. Can chair yoga actually boost energy in older adults?

Certainly! The mix of attentive movement, breathing, and meditation in chair yoga adds to greater vitality, supporting a more lively and active existence.

3. How often should elders practice chair yoga for maximum vitality?

Seniors might benefit from practicing chair yoga 2-3 times a week for maximum health. Consistency is crucial to obtaining enduring results.

4. Can chair yoga be performed by seniors with restricted mobility?

Yes, chair yoga is very adjustable, making it suited for seniors with various levels of mobility. Poses can be changed to fit specific requirements.

5. What sets Access Health Care Physicians, LLC's chair yoga classes apart?

Access Health treatment Physicians, LLC's chair yoga sessions are part of a holistic approach to senior health, incorporating professional supervision and tailored treatment to boost vitality and general well-being.

Embark on a journey to vibrant senior living with Yoga for Seniors in a Chair, presented to you by Access Health Care Physicians, LLC, where each position is a step towards a more alive and enriched existence.

Chapter 1

DISCOVERING CHAIR YOGA

What is Chair Yoga?

Chair yoga is a moderate style of yoga that's done while seated or utilizing a chair for balance, making the practice more accessible. In chair yoga, it's possible to go into positions like cat/cow, warrior, sun salutations, and forward folds, all while seated.

Kelly feels the Arthur Ashe motto, "Start where you are, use what you have, do what you can," is excellent for chair yoga.

"You're there to work and to challenge yourself, but it about knows what's right for you," she adds. "I believe yoga poses should be adapted to fit a student's body, rather than forcing the body to conform to the poses."

Whether yoga is done in a chair or on the mat, the practice still focuses on the same key principles: focusing on your breath, paying attention to your thoughts, and remaining in the now.

What are the benefits of Chair Yoga?

There are hundreds of benefits of doing Chair Yoga this helps in the:

1. **Improved flexibility and mobility:** Chair yoga contains mild stretches and motions that assist improve joint flexibility, increasing range of motion, and enhancing general mobility. It can assist elders in maintaining and developing their physical abilities while reducing stiffness and tightness in the body.

2. **Strength building:** Chair yoga involves sitting poses and mild resistance exercises that help seniors develop their muscles. Regular practice can lead to increased muscular tone, stability, and balance, minimizing the chance of falls and accidents.

3. **Enhanced posture and alignment:** Sitting for extended durations can lead to poor posture and alignment concerns. Chair yoga focuses on perfect posture, encouraging seniors to sit tall and utilize their core muscles. This helps improve posture and lowers pressure on the back and neck.

4. **Stress reduction and relaxation:** Chair yoga involves breathing techniques and meditation, giving seniors tools to manage stress, and anxiety, and promote relaxation. Deep

breathing exercises can help relax the mind, increase attention, and reduce tension.

5. **Increased energy and vitality:** Gentle movements and stretches in chair yoga assist improve circulation, enhance the body's energy flow, and promote overall vitality. Seniors may feel greater energy levels, better mood, and a sense of well-being.

6. **Social engagement and community:** Participating in chair yoga courses helps seniors to engage with others, promoting a feeling of community and social interaction. This can battle feelings of loneliness and create a supportive setting for sharing experiences and creating connections.

Who should try Chair Yoga?

Although chair yoga is generally recommended as a practice for people who may struggle with mat practice, anybody may benefit from this form of gentle exercise.

Kelly believes chair yoga is particularly well-suited to persons who use wheelchairs and those rehabbing after surgeries, living with chronic diseases, or coping with balance challenges that make it hard to go down onto a yoga mat. It's also excellent for a fast workout during the workday or while traveling.

"It's not about the outcome. It's not about achieving the ideal pose," Kelly says. ""Whether yoga is practiced on a mat or in a chair, it's all about maintaining good health."

Chair yoga is particularly perfect for beginners who might be intimidated by a typical mat practice since it gives a safe approach to learning the poses.

How to Get Started

To practice at home, use a sturdy chair (an office chair on wheels or an overstuffed armchair is not suitable for chair yoga). Minard offers a chair that naturally sets your hips slightly higher than your knees and allows you to put both feet flat on the floor.

"If your feet aren't flat on the ground, your weight is concentrated in your spine, and if the chair is too low with your knees above your hips, there is more impingement on your hips," Minard adds. "You aim to perform slow, controlled movements without placing additional strain on your back or hips."

Make sure the chair is on a solid surface like a carpet or a yoga mat to protect it from slipping. You can even prop the back of the chair against a wall for added support, Minard says.

Yoga props like blocks, harnesses, and resistance bands that are typical in mat practices aren't necessary for chair yoga -- unless you want an added challenge.

"Chair yoga is an excellent way to engage muscles that may not have been used recently, minimizing the risk of overloading your muscles and joints or falling," Minard explains. "If the resistance from your body weight is insufficient, you can enhance your chair yoga practice by incorporating light hand weights, ankle weights, or resistance bands."

Yoga Myths Debunked: 10 Common Misconceptions About Yoga Explained

Yoga is a technique that has been mired in myths and misconceptions for millennia. From misconceptions about who may practice yoga to what it requires, these falsehoods can frequently dissuade individuals from enjoying the transforming benefits of yoga. In this tutorial, we'll dispel 10 common myths about yoga, bringing clarity and knowledge about what yoga is and who may benefit from it. By refuting these stereotypes, we seek to make yoga more accessible and inclusive for everyone.

Myth: Yoga is only for the flexible.

- **Reality:** One of the most popular misunderstandings about yoga is that it's only for the flexible. In actuality, yoga is for everyone, regardless of age, body shape, or fitness level. Yoga is a discipline of self-discovery and self-acceptance, and there are adaptations and variants for every position to suit varied levels of flexibility.

Myth: Yoga is merely stretching.

- **Reality:** While yoga does include stretching, it's much more than just that. Yoga is a comprehensive practice that incorporates breath, movement, mindfulness, and meditation to enhance physical, mental, and emotional well-being. Yoga also increases strength, balance, and flexibility, while soothing the mind and lowering stress.

Myth: Yoga is only for women.

- **Reality:** While yoga has historically been done largely by women, it is not solely for either gender. Men, women, and persons of all gender identities can benefit from the practice of yoga. In reality, many elite athletes, military people, and business leaders include yoga in their workout routines.

Myth: You have to be spiritual or religious to do yoga.

- **Reality:** While yoga has origins in old spiritual traditions, it is neither necessarily religious nor spiritual. Yoga can be done as a merely physical exercise or as a spiritual journey, depending on individual beliefs and inclinations. Many people feel that yoga strengthens their spiritual connection or develops their current spirituality, although it is not necessary for practice.

Myth: You need costly yoga clothes and equipment to perform yoga.

- **Reality:** One of the charms of yoga is its simplicity and accessibility. You don't need sophisticated yoga attire or expensive equipment to do yoga—all you need is a comfortable outfit and a yoga mat. While props like blocks, straps, and blankets might help your practice, they are not needed.

Myth: Yoga is only for young people.

- **Reality:** Yoga is for people of all ages, from children to elders. Yoga can be particularly good for older persons, since it develops flexibility, mobility, balance, and strength, while also lowering the risk of falls and accidents. There are various gentle and chair yoga courses particularly suited for elders.

Myth: You have to be slim to do yoga.

- **Reality:** Yoga is for bodies of all shapes and sizes. It's not about how you appear in a stance, but how you feel in your body and mind. Yoga is a discipline of self-acceptance and self-love, and everybody is capable of enjoying the benefits of yoga, regardless of size or form.

Myth: You need to be in good physical condition to practice yoga.

- **Reality:** Yoga is a practice that meets you where you are, regardless of your present fitness level. Whether you're a novice or an expert yogi, there are classes and types of yoga that suit your needs and talents. Yoga is about development, not perfection, and every practice is a chance for growth and self-discovery.

Myth: Yoga is too slow and boring.

- **Reality:** While certain kinds of yoga may be slower-paced, many dynamic and hard styles of yoga deliver a powerful exercise. From power yoga to vinyasa flow, some courses will have your pulse racing and your body sweating. Plus, yoga is anything from boring—each practice is a voyage of investigation and self-discovery.

Myth: You have to be able to touch your toes to practice yoga.

- **Reality:** Yoga is not about reaching your toes or attaining a perfect pose—it's about the path of self-discovery and self-improvement. Everybody is distinct, and every practice is unique. The beauty of yoga comes in the process of inquiry and progress, not in obtaining a particular conclusion.

Conclusion

Yoga is a discipline that has been shrouded by myths and misconceptions for far too long. By refuting some common beliefs about yoga, we seek to make yoga more accessible, inclusive, and welcoming for everyone. Whether you're young or old, supple or stiff, spiritual or secular, there is a place for you in the world of yoga. So let go of your assumptions, lay out your mat, and explore the transformational power of yoga for yourself.

Chapter 2

PREPARING FOR YOUR JOURNEY

What are the precautions before performing yoga?

Five Essential Tips to Know Before Beginning Yoga:

1. Patience is the key to being successful:

This is the first thing that a person must learn. Yoga does not provide effects in one day. You have to practice frequently for at least 30 to 45 days, with uttermost devotion to envision outcomes. Be it for weight reduction, weight gain, or diabetes, frequent indulgence in yoga is likely to bring you results, but time is the watchword.

2. Always practice yoga in serenity:

A silent setting is the primary need for doing yoga. The room should be airy as well. You can turn on some light music, particularly mantras such as Om. Silence and calm will help you concentrate on your asanas and breathing, therefore equipping you with the capacity to listen and accept your body's requirements in a very pleasant way. Every breath you take should be kept track of.

That is one of the primary reasons why gurus encourage you to practice yoga early in the morning or evening. This is when the surroundings will be free of sounds, therefore allowing you to know your inner self totally and alter yourself.

3. Always wear comfy apparel:

Always pick attire in which you feel comfortable. Loose, comfortable garments will assist you breathe well while executing the asanas. Tight garments might hinder free mobility and at times even result in injury. Choose cotton garments, ideally a tee and loose track trousers, since these enable absorption of the perspiration and let you practice your asanas with total focus.

4. Never eat a large meal shortly before your yoga practice:

As with other fitness regimes, yoga also does not enable you to perform with a full stomach. Try to practice yoga early in the morning, half an hour after a cup of coffee. If that does not suit you, then make sure that you wait for at least two hours after breakfast and four hours after lunch, before doing yoga. There are quite a lot of asanas that focus on the abdomen. Working out on a full stomach might give unpleasant outcomes while performing those stances.

5. An instructor is necessary to learn yoga properly.

There are several websites now that give A to Z information concerning the different styles of yoga, asanas, and much more. However, if you are new to yoga, then it is important to seek the presence of a trainer yogin or yogini [yoga teacher], who can teach you the appropriate manner of executing asanas. Like other exercises, even the tiniest error while practicing an asana might result in damage. Hence, the presence of a guru is of the biggest significance.

What are the physical activities for older citizens?

Chair Tai Chi

Similar to chair yoga, chair Tai Chi modifies conventional Tai Chi techniques for sitting individuals. Tai Chi focuses on gentle, flowing motions that promote balance, strength, and relaxation. Seniors in memory care might benefit from performing Tai Chi practices meant to increase physical stability and mental clarity, generating a sense of peace and well-being.

Indoor Gardening

Indoor gardening offers seniors with a therapeutic and meaningful pastime that stimulates their senses and promotes physical exercise. Memory care users can engage in planting, watering, and caring for indoor plants or small herb gardens. Gardening activities allow light movement, sensory stimulation, and a sense of accomplishment as plants grow and thrive.

Adaptive Sports

Memory care facilities can offer adapted sports programs customized to elders' skills and interests. Activities such as modified bowling, bocce ball, or shuffleboard give possibilities for friendly competition, hand-eye coordination, and physical activity. These sports may be customized with equipment and regulations to meet differing skill levels and mobility restrictions.

Stretching Circles

Stretching circles are group activities led by teachers or staff members, concentrating on mild stretching and flexibility exercises. Seniors sit in a circle and follow along with guided stretches targeting different muscle areas. Stretching circles promote flexibility, reduce stiffness, and boost circulation, increasing general physical comfort and well-being.

Sensory Stations

Sensory stations are interactive sets meant to excite the senses through various activities and materials. Memory care seniors can engage in sensory activities such as tactile stimulation with textured items, aromatherapy with fragrant oils, or auditory stimulation with relaxing music or natural sounds. These exercises enhance calm, sensory awareness, and emotional management.

Balloon Toss

Balloon throw is a simple yet entertaining sport that enables seniors to engage in modest physical exercise and social contact. Residents form a circle and carefully toss a soft balloon to each other, hoping to keep it aloft without letting it strike the ground. Balloon toss increases hand-eye coordination, laughing, and camaraderie among players, promoting a sense of connection and pleasure.

Conclusion

Incorporating a broad range of physical workouts adapted to the requirements and capabilities of seniors in memory care facilities at senior living homes in Frisco, TX, is crucial for promoting their physical and mental well-being. These 10 suggested exercises give a variety of advantages, such as strengthening strength and flexibility, encouraging balance, and improving cognitive function. Seeking help from healthcare specialists or fitness experts is vital in establishing a specific workout routine.

How much exercise do you need if you are older than 70?

Before you start ANY activity, check with your doctor to be sure it is appropriate for you.

Several individuals have addressed the necessity of cardio-type exercises.

Daily walking is a good concept for older adults. It takes no equipment and can be done practically any place.

Can't get out?

Walk in place to some energetic music. Get a companion and stroll the corridors in your apartment or condo complex.

Unsteady on your feet?

Sit in a chair and march in place.

Having said, all that, I'd want to focus on safety.

One of the greatest concerns of elderly individuals is falls. Many individuals, once they fall, can't get back up.

If you live alone this can be dangerous.

I could regale you with stories of persons "found down" who were unable to receive treatment and later died. Many were found dehydrated, in their excrement and urine, after resting on the floor for days.

Here is the test I used with elderly folks.

I would instruct them to take a seat on the floor.

Then I would have them try to stand up, without help. They could crawl or scoot but they had to do it, alone.

It was genuinely eye-opening, to many individuals, that they couldn't do so.

If that's the case, a very honest talk has to ensue regarding physical therapy and the wisdom of living alone.

This talent might be the difference between living in your house and your kids losing their collective sh*t and asking that you go to a facility.

So, what do you do?

Strength, flexibility, and balance are the critical components in keeping on your feet.

Activities like weight training, starting slowly and at a level appropriate for your present level of fitness, are highly significant. Progress slowly to avoid harm.

Older adults lose muscle at a frightening pace if they don't work on this. You would be astonished at how fast you lose it if you don't utilize it.

A physical therapist or personal trainer can help initiate your journey.

Flexibility and balance are the two things elderly people tend to forget about.

If you can't adjust to varied surfaces, have rigid joints, or have constraints to your movement, even small ones, you will go down like a tree when challenged. (Think "Timber!")

Improving your flexibility and balance can be attained through Tai Chi, yoga, or stretching.

You don't have to be a Spandex Princess or stretch yourself into a pretzel. There are several classes for Seniors, such as Chair Yoga and Seated Tai Chi.

Try your local senior center or YMCA.

It's tough for some Seniors to get out in inclement weather. DVDs are available for home use.

The objective is consistency.

Have a program that you do most days of the week. Changing things up a bit.

Walk one day, weights the next. Sneak in some stretching before you get out of bed. Stand on one foot, then the other as you clean your teeth or wait for the coffee to make.

Go to a yoga class. Put on a video. Stay involved with others. Measure your progress.

This helps to fight off boredom and keep you engaged.

However, above all, consult with your doctor first.

Your level of fitness at 70 may very well influence where you spend the remainder of your life.

Chapter 3

THE ESSENTIALS OF CHAIR YOGA

What are the 6 yoga positions for beginners?

Here are six yoga positions that are perfect for beginners:

Mountain Pose (Tadasana):

Stand tall with your feet hip-width apart, press down through your feet, extend your spine, and relax your shoulders. This pose helps to enhance posture and promote awareness of the body.

Downward-Facing Dog (Adho Mukha Svanasana):

Begin on your hands and knees, with your wrists precisely under your shoulders and your knees under your hips. Exhale and pull your hips up and back, straightening your arms and legs. This position helps to stretch and strengthen the entire body.

Warrior I (Virabhadrasana I):

From a downward-facing dog, step your right foot forward between your hands. Turn your left foot out to a 45-degree angle and push down through the outside edge of your foot. Inhale and extend your arms up overhead. This position helps to strengthen the legs and enhance balance.

Triangle Pose (Trikonasana):

From Warrior I, extend your front leg and raise your right hand forward as far as you can. Then, hinge at your hip and bring your right hand down towards your shin or the floor. Reach your left arm up towards the ceiling. This position helps to stretch the hamstrings and hips, while also strengthening the legs.

Tree Pose (Vrikshasana):

Stand upright with your feet close together. Transfer your weight onto your left foot and lift your right foot off the ground. Position the sole of your right foot against your left inner thigh, press it gently into your thigh, and maintain balance on your left foot. Bring your hands together at your heart or stretch them aloft. This stance helps to enhance balance and attention.

Child's Pose (Balasana):

Position yourself on the floor with your knees spaced hip-width apart and toes touching. Sit back on your heels and fold forward, putting your forehead on the floor. Reach your arms out in front of you or rest them alongside your body. This position helps to alleviate tension in the neck, shoulders, and back, while also fostering relaxation.

Remember to always listen to your body and adjust or skip postures that don't feel comfortable for you. It's crucial to move gently and thoughtfully as you explore these yoga positions.

What are some breathing methods used in yoga, and what are their benefits?

Breathing is a crucial process that starts at the moment of birth and ceases only when a person dies. Each breathing cycle comprises the intake of life-sustaining oxygen to give to all organs and cells of the body and the throwing out of carbon dioxide (toxin) from inside.

Look at the following table to see how the pace of breathing is connected to the life duration of humans and various animals. We might draw from this data that, "breathless to live longer" or in other words "live fast and die young"

Animal	Breath per minute	Average age (Year)
Tortoise	3 – 4	200+
Human	12 – 15	70+
Horse	15 – 18	40

Goat	18	16
Dog	22	12
Mouse	160	1 – 2

The table diagram lets us grasp the many sorts of breathing and how to make maximum out of it to breathe less to live longer and healthier.

Our breathing area is separated into three different portions dependent on the section of the body and lungs space we utilize to breathe.

Abdominal breathing - Here, as we breathe in, the lungs expand, and the diaphragm (organ below the lungs) glides down and pushes the abdominal organs outwards (essentially, the belly bulges like a balloon). This makes use of the abdominal region of the lungs to store oxygen. Abdominal breathing optimizes the lung capacity and makes breathing rhythmic and calming,

Thoracic breathing - Here, we make use of the thoracic area of the lungs to breathe, and thus, as we breathe chest region expands and goes back as we breathe out. It is a fast kind of breathing that causes a heightened sense of tension.

Clavicular breathing - Here we make use of the top region of the lungs, above the chest level. In this kind, the breathing is very shallow and quick and it happens in moments of high stress and fear, or when there is considerable difficulty in breathing.

Observe a freshly born newborn breathing and observe how the tummy bulges out and goes back and that is what abdominal breathing, is suggested for a good life.

So, when do we move from abdominal breathing to thoracic breathing? That is generally occurring when we are in fight or flight mode. next time notice your breathing pattern, when you are asleep, and when you are in some stress, worried, or furious mode, you will note the difference. And, both patterns of breathing are required according to situations but, in recent days, with changes in human lifestyle, people end up spending most of their time in stressful situations and that makes thoracic breathing more than abdominal breathing and so we tend to follow shallow and fast breathing during most of our day.

Yogic breathing incorporates all the three forms of breathing discussed above optimizes the lung capacity and makes the breathing deep, rhythmic, and soothing.

One typical error individuals do is, sucking in the belly or abdomen during breathing in as the chest expands, instead of bulging the belly or releasing the abdomen forward.

Pranayama (combination of 2 words: prana - the essential energy for life and ayama - by stretching or expanding), the 4th anga (part) of guru Patanjali's yoga sutras, is a discipline of controlling and regulating the breath.

Why is breathing vital whilst practicing yoga?

Breathing is incredibly crucial in yoga, just like it is in everyday life. Think of it as the secret sauce that helps everything in yoga operate better. When you're performing yoga, breathing appropriately helps you move smoother, feel stronger, and stay calm.

Imagine attempting to fill a balloon while squeezing the entrance a bit. It's going to fill up slowly and not as well, right? That's kind of what happens when you don't breathe properly during yoga. You're not providing your body with all the excellent stuff it needs to accomplish its best.

But when you breathe deeply and in sync with your motions, it's like opening that balloon all the way. Your body becomes loaded with energy, your muscles operate better, and your mind stays cool and collected. It's like gaining a power-up in a video game.

Not breathing appropriately, or holding your air, is like attempting to sprint with one shoe on. Sure, you can still move, but you won't go as swiftly or as smoothly as you might. Breathing appropriately helps everything in yoga seem easier and more effective.

Plus, focusing on your breath may make you feel calmer and serene, not just during yoga but at other times of your day too. It's a method to settle down when things become frantic and to feel more alert and alive when you're exhausted.

So, in yoga, breathing isn't just a minor thing; it's everything. It helps you stretch further, hold postures longer, and feel better while doing it. Remember, breathe deep, and let the magic happen!

Chapter 4

WEEK 1 - BUILDING STRENGTH

Day 1-3: What are the greatest yoga positions for core strength?

In the quest for general fitness and well-being, a strong core is typically considered the cornerstone. Beyond cosmetic benefits, a firm core adds to stability, balance, and increased functional mobility. Yoga, with its holistic approach to physical and mental well-being, provides a plethora of postures that especially target and strengthen the core. Let's go into the realm of yoga and unearth some of the greatest positions to spark and build your core strength.

Try these positions 2 times while practicing yoga. Please warm up first before starting.

Plank Pose (Phalakasana)

Begin in a push-up stance, ensuring your wrists are directly aligned under your shoulders. Keep your body in a straight line from head to heels, activating your core muscles. Hold the posture for 30 seconds to a minute, or longer as you increase strength.

Boat Pose (Navasana)

Sit on the floor, lean back slightly, and elevate your legs, making a V shape with your torso. Keep your back straight and stretch your arms parallel to the floor. This position targets the abdominal muscles, helping to increase strength and endurance.

Downward-Facing Dog (Adho Mukha Svanasana)

Begin on your hands and knees, tuck your toes, and elevate your hips toward the ceiling, producing an inverted V shape. This position utilizes the entire body, including the core, while also extending and strengthening the back.

Side Plank (Vasisthasana)

From plank posture, move your weight onto one hand and twist your body, stacking your feet on top of each other. Raise your upper arm toward the ceiling. This position emphasizes the obliques and promotes lateral strength.

Bridge Pose (Setu Bandhasana)

Rest on your back, bend your knees, and align your feet hip-width apart. Press through your feet to elevate your hips toward the ceiling. This position works the core, glutes, and lower back, developing strength and flexibility.

Warrior III (Virabhadrasana III)

From a standing posture, shift your weight onto one leg and stretch the other leg behind you, parallel to the floor. Simultaneously, stretch your arms forward. This posture stresses the core's stability and promotes general balance.

Leg Raises

Lie on your back and elevate your legs toward the ceiling, maintaining them straight. Lower them carefully toward the floor without letting them contact. This workout targets the lower abdominal muscles, developing strength and tone.

Chair Pose (Utkatasana)

Stand with your feet together, bend your knees, and drop your hips as if you are sitting in an imagined chair. This posture stimulates the whole core, especially the muscles surrounding the spine.

Day 4-7: Focus on Core Stability

Here are some excellent chair yoga postures for core strength, along with a brief description of their advantages and step-by-step directions on how to practice them:

Seated Twist

This position emphasizes the oblique's and deep spinal muscles, enhancing spinal mobility and core strength.

1. Sit up tall on a chair with your feet flat on the floor.
2. Place your right hand on your left knee and your left hand on the back of the chair or the seat behind you.
3. Inhale deeply and stretch your spine; as you exhale, slowly twist to the left, using your hands for leverage.
4. Hold the twist for 3-5 breaths, then return to the center and repeat on the other side.

Seated Cat-Cow

This position works the deep core muscles and increases spinal flexibility.

1. Sit up tall in a chair with your feet flat on the floor and your hands resting on your knees.
2. Inhale and arch your back, elevate your chest, and gaze upward for Cow posture.
3. Exhale and circle your back, tucking your chin against your chest and pulling your navel near your spine for Cat posture.
4. Continue alternating between Cat and Cow positions for 5-10 breaths.

Seated Leg Lifts

This position strengthens the hip flexors and lower abdominals, enhancing core stability and balance.

1. Sit up straight in a chair with your feet flat on the floor and your hands resting on your thighs or holding onto the edges of the chair for support.
2. Engage your core and slowly pull your right leg toward your chest while keeping your spine straight and tall.
3. Hold the leg raise for 2-3 breaths, then slowly drop your foot back to the floor.
4. Repeat with the left leg and continue alternating legs for 5-10 repetitions on each side.

Seated Boat Pose

This position emphasizes the lower abdominals, hip flexors, and lower back muscles, strengthening core stability and balance.

1. Sit on the edge of a chair with your feet flat on the floor and your hands holding onto the edges of the chair for support.
2. Lean back slightly and engage your core, bringing your feet off the floor while maintaining your knees bent.
3. Hold this posture for 5-10 breaths, maintaining a straight spine and steady core throughout.

4. Gently drop your feet back to the floor and release.

Seated Side Bend

This position works the obliques and helps improve total core strength and flexibility.

1. Sit up tall on a chair with your feet flat on the floor and your arms at your sides.
2. Inhale and stretch your right arm above, lengthening your spine.
3. Exhale and bend your body to the left, keeping your right arm extended and your left hand resting on your left thigh or the seat of the chair.
4. Hold the side bend for 3-5 breaths, then return to the center and repeat on the other side.

Seated Pike Pulse

This position strengthens the whole core, including the abdominals, obliques, and lower back muscles.

1. Sit on the edge of a chair with your legs stretched in front of you and your heels resting on the floor.
2. Place your hands on your thighs or hang onto the edges of the chair for support.

3. Engage your core and elevate your chest, keeping a straight spine.

4. Inhale and lean back slightly, then exhale and pulse forward, contracting your abdominals as if attempting to touch your toes.

5. Continue pulsating for 10-15 repetitions, keeping your core engaged and your spine straight.

Conclusion

The definitive guide to chair yoga for core strength gives significant insights into the advantages and mechanics of Chair yoga for increasing core strength. By adopting a range of positions that target different core muscles, individuals may enhance their stability, balance, and general well-being.

Chair yoga offers an accessible and low-impact technique to strengthen core strength, appealing to people of all ages and fitness levels. Embrace this transforming practice and discover the great influence it may have on your everyday life.

Day 7: Review and Reflect: Progress and Adjustments

Reflection Questions:

1. What have you done thus far? Acknowledge your successes, no matter how small they might seem.

2. What challenges have you experienced, and how have you overcome them?

3. What modifications do you need to make to keep on track or overcome any remaining obstacles?

4. What habits or routines are functioning well for you, and which ones require refinement?

5. How has your thinking or approach towards your goals altered since starting this journey?

6. Are there any places where you feel trapped or frustrated? What can you do to address these feelings and move forward?

Adjustments and Refining Your Approach:

Based on your reflection, identify areas where you need to make modifications to keep on course or overcome problems. Consider the following:

1. Refine your objectives: Are there any particular goals that need rephrasing or re-evaluation? Make sure your goals are still aligned with your beliefs and priorities.

2. Adjust your routine: Are there any habits or routines that aren't serving you well? Make modifications to enhance your everyday routine for increased productivity and efficiency.

3. Seek support: Are there any resources or individuals who could assist you overcome problems or stay motivated? Seek assistance from friends, family, or professionals.

4. Appreciate tiny wins: Acknowledge and appreciate the small accomplishments along the road. This will help you stay inspired and encouraged to continue working towards your goals.

5. Practice self-care: Don't forget to prioritize self-care and take breaks when required. A revitalized mind and body can help you confront obstacles more successfully.

Remember, it's natural to suffer setbacks or changes along the route. The idea is to learn from them and change accordingly.

Action Plan for the Next 7 Days:

1. Continue monitoring progress: Keep a diary or record to monitor your progress and reflect on what's going well.

2. Adjust habits and routines: Implement changes depending on your thoughts and modifications needed.

3. Seek support: Reach out to individuals or services that can help you stay motivated and conquer problems.

4. Appreciate tiny wins: Acknowledge and appreciate the small accomplishments along the road.

5. Prioritize self-care: Make time for rest, relaxation, and self-care activities.

By reflecting on your accomplishments and making any modifications, you'll be better ready to tackle the following 7 days with confidence and enthusiasm.

Remember

Consistency is crucial, but it's also necessary to be adaptable and adjust to changing situations. Stay focused, motivated, and devoted to your goals, and you'll be celebrating your triumphs in no time!

Chapter 5

WEEK 2 - ENHANCING FLEXIBILITY

Day 8-10: excellent workouts and stretches for lower back

5 Easy Stretches to Alleviate Lower Back Pain

Kneeling Lunge Stretch

- Start by kneeling on both knees and moving one leg forward until the foot is flat on the ground.
- Ensure that your weight is evenly distributed over both hips, rather than favoring one side.
- Lean forward, placing both hands on the top of your thigh, to feel a stretch in the front of the opposite leg.
- This stretch targets the hip flexor muscles, which are vital for maintaining excellent posture.

Piriformis Muscle Stretch

- Lie on your back with your knees bent and your heels resting flat on the floor.

- Cross one leg over the other, resting the ankle on the bent knee, and gently bring the lower knee towards your chest to feel a stretch in the buttock.

- Alternatively, lie on the floor and cross one leg over the other, pushing it forward over the body at the knee while maintaining the other leg flat.

Cobra Stretch

- This stretch is good for stretching tight abdominal muscles and the lower back.

- Begin by laying on your stomach, legs outstretched, palms placed on each side of your head, forearms and elbows flat on the ground.

- Slowly elevate your body such that your weight is supported on your forearms.

- Ensure that your hips remain firmly planted on the ground.

- Hold for 10 seconds, progressively stretching your abdominal muscles and lower back.

- Slowly return to the beginning position and repeat five times.

- If you have greater flexibility in your lower back, straighten your arms during the stretch.

Child's Pose

- The calming Child's Pose, a foundational yoga pose, can assist in the relaxation of the body.
- Begin by situating yourself on the floor on your hands and knees, with knees slightly wider than hip-width apart.
- Bring your toes together and softly press your hips back while bending your knees.
- Find a comfortable sitting position, completely stretching your arms forward and allowing your head to relax forward.
- Maintain this posture for 20 seconds before returning to the beginning position and repeating three more times.
- If you have soreness in your shoulders, lay your arms beside your body and reach them towards your feet.

Sitting Spinal Twist

- An easy sitting spinal twist helps ease lower back discomfort and promote flexibility.
- This easy stretch delivers various health advantages, including increased happiness and flexibility in the knees, spine, and shoulders.
- Sit on the floor with legs outstretched in front of you and arms behind your back.

- Place both hands on the floor behind you, with your fingers pointing away from your body.
- Plant your left foot flat on the ground outside of your right knee.
- Inhale as you lift your right arm.
- Exhale as you bring your right arm down, resting your elbow on the outside of your left leg.
- Rotate your chest, head, and eyeballs to the left.
- Hold for roughly one minute, inhaling deeply. Slowly bring your head and chest to the middle.
- Repeat on the opposite side.

Note: Are you weary of living with persistent discomfort from sciatica, piriformis syndrome, hip pain, SI joint pain, and more? Say goodbye to your suffering with the Acu-Hump Sciatica Stretcher. This unique massage tool is particularly successful in delivering treatment for a range of unpleasant situations.

The Acu-Hump Sciatica Stretcher is uniquely developed to target and ease pain in the hip, buttocks, and back. Its deep tissue massage effect helps to reduce tension and offer relief for sciatic nerve discomfort. You may apply it from your lower back down to your hips for optimum effect.

Day 11-13: Stretching the Upper Body Yoga poses and stretches

The following upper-body exercises can be done simultaneously or one at a time throughout your day. They assist you focus on the places where you feel tight. With each posture or stretch, keep a deep and steady breath. Hold each posture for 30 to 60 seconds or longer. Don't strain or produce discomfort; let each position gradually stretch and remove stiffness.

Neck release

- Tuck your chin (create a double chin).
- Roll your chin toward your chest. Create a stretch behind your head and hold.
- Keep your chin tucked. Look to the right and hold. Look to the left and hold.

Hand, wrist, and elbow rescue

- Hands: Facepalms facing each other, with your fingers touching. Stretch your fingers apart. Press your palms toward each other to stretch the areas between and behind your fingers.
- Wrist/elbow: Reach your right arm forward, palm turned upward with your elbow straight. Reach out with your left

arm, connect your palms, and press your right fingers toward the floor. Repeat on the opposite side.

Torso, back, and shoulder flow

- Interlace your fingers. Rotate your palms outward from your body. Breathe in. Straighten your arms. Press your hands forward and stretch your torso forward. Lift your body erect and hands overhead. Exhale—arms drift down to sides.
- Repeat the above three to five times.

Last time

Torso and shoulder release: Hold your arms above your head, fingers intertwined, and palms toward the sky. Press upward via your palms. Stretch across the front of shoulders and chest, and hold.

Upper back opener

Reach arms forward, pressing palms forward. Round upper back, tuck in chin. Move hands from side to side. Stretch behind and between shoulder blades, and hold.

Energizing backbend, chest opener

Place hands on hips or lower back. Inhale, raising your chest high.

Look up. Pull your elbows back. Open your shoulders, extend your chest, and hold.

Spinal stretch

- Place your feet 12 to 18 inches apart. Inhale, arms up. Exhale, round your torso forward. Rest your forearms on your thighs. Let your spine round. Relax your head and neck, and hold.
- Inhale, draw abdominal muscles in. Slowly roll up. Stretch arms upwards, exhale, and return hands to lap.

Half-moon – side bend

- Inhale, stretch left arm up, right arm down. Lift and extend the spine. Exhale, bend your torso toward the right; keep your shoulders square, and hold.
- Repeat on the left side.

Soothing sitting twist

- Inhale, arms up. Exhale and move the body to the right—place left hand on the right knee—right hand to seat or back of the chair. Inhale sit tall—exhale open the chest—broaden the shoulders—and hold.
- Repeat on the left side.

Progressive muscle relaxation for the upper body: The act of tightening and releasing your muscles helps you become aware of any muscular tension. Tension may intensify stress, which can raise muscular tension even higher. Use this approach to help break the stress-tension cycle and to relax at any time. For this technique:

- Sit back in your chair with a tall spine.
- Reach your arms forward. Make a fist. Engage your arms, chest, upper back, shoulders, jaw, and forehead. Pause and observe how your stiff, constricted muscles feel.
- Inhale gently and deeply. Exhale very gently; gradually drop your hands to your lap.
- Continue to breathe deeply.
- Release palms to your lap—spread your fingers. Allow arms to dangle heavily from the shoulders into your hands.
- Relieve tension in the upper back, shoulders, and chest.
- Allow your forehead to soften and your jaw to loosen. Relax your entire face.
- Repeat three to five times or until you feel free of stress.
- Continue to breathe deeply—scan your body for leftover traces of tightness to soften and release the tension.

Yoga relaxation – Savasana

- Lean back in your chair, close your eyes, and let your hands rest in your lap.
- Allow your breath to return to a regular light and effortless rhythm. Continue to examine your breath—follow and feel the inhales and exhales.
- Observe your body—release residual tension.
- Allow a sensation of effortlessness, well-being, and calm to move through your body.
- Let your thinking feel light and quiet—just like the breath.
- Sit quietly for one to five minutes or until you feel calm and rejuvenated.

Day 14: Review and Reflect: Flexibility Gains

Reflection Questions:

1. How has your flexibility increased since commencing your daily stretching routine? Have you seen any notable alterations in your range of motion or ease of movement?
2. Which stretches have been the most tough for you, and how have you overcome those challenges?
3. Have you noticed any physical or mental advantages from implementing flexibility exercises into your everyday

routine? (e.g., decreased stiffness, improved posture, more energy)

4. What are some frequent hurdles you've met when stretching, and how have you overcome them? (e.g., lack of motivation, pain, tiredness)

5. How has adding flexibility exercises influenced your entire lifestyle and daily activities? (e.g., better mobility, lower injury risk, greater sports performance)

Reviewing Your Progress:

Take time to think about the stretches you've been doing each day and note any improvements you've seen in your flexibility. Ask yourself:

- Are there any areas where you've experienced considerable improvement?

- Are there any stretches that still feel tough or uncomfortable? Why would that be?

- Have you observed any trends or correlations between various stretches and certain muscle groups or regions of tension?

Tips for Continued Progress:

1. Listen to your body: If you're feeling exhausted or suffering discomfort during stretches, take a break or alter the stretch to make it more pleasant.

2. Focus on consistency: Aim to maintain stretching consistently, even if it's just a few minutes a day. Consistency is crucial to establishing flexibility.

3. Experiment with different stretches: Try new stretches or variations to keep your practice fresh and challenging.

4. Combine with other exercises: Incorporate strength training or other types of exercise to increase the advantages of flexibility training.

5. Make it a habit: Incorporate stretching into your everyday routine, such as shortly after waking up or before bed.

Next Steps:

1. Continue with your regular stretching program and make modifications as required.

2. Gradually increase the time or intensity of your stretches as you grow more comfortable.

3. Experiment with different stretches or exercises to keep your program fresh and challenging.

4. Consider combining other kinds of exercise, such as yoga or Pilates, to complement your flexibility training.

Remember, flexibility is a journey, and development may be gradual and steady. Be patient, keep consistent, and enjoy tiny triumphs along the road!

Chapter 6

WEEK 3 - MASTERING BALANCE

Day 15-17: Simple Balancing Exercises

These workouts are available to all levels.

1. Rock the boat

- Stand with your feet hip-distance apart.
- Raise your arms and stretch them outward to each side.
- Lift your left foot off the floor and bend your knee to move your heel closer to your bottom.
- Maintain this posture for a maximum of 30 seconds.
- Then do the opposite side.
- Do each side 3 repetitions.

2. Weight shifts

- Stand with your feet hip-width apart.
- Shift your weight onto your right foot.
- Raise your left foot.
- Maintain this posture for a maximum of 30 seconds.
- Then do the opposite side.

- Do each side 3 repetitions.
- Core exercises

3. Tightrope walk

This easy workout improves balance, posture, and core strength.

- Extend your arms and raise them out to the sides.
- Walk in a straight path while fixing your sight on a specific object in the distance.
- Each time you elevate your foot, pause with your foot in this raised posture for 2 to 3 seconds.
- Take 20 to 30 steps.

4. Flamingo stand

- Shift your weight onto your right foot.
- Lift your left foot and stretch your leg forward.
- Hold this position for 10 to 15 seconds.
- Increase the difficulty by stretching your hands toward your outstretched foot.
- Return to the starting posture and shake off your legs.
- Repeat 3 times.
- Then do the opposite side.
- Posture exercises

5. Back leg lifts

This exercise strengthens your lower back and glutes, which helps promote excellent posture.

- Place your hands against a wall or the back of a chair.
- Shift your weight onto your right foot.
- Slowly pull your left leg back and up as high as you can.
- Hold this posture for 5 seconds.
- Return to the starting position.
- Do 10 repetitions.
- Then do the opposite side.
- Balance and strength workouts

6. Tree posture

During this exercise, refrain from placing your foot on your knee.

- Shift your weight onto your right foot from a standing position.
- Position your left foot to the side with your heel elevated, or put the sole of your foot on your ankle, shin, or thigh.
- Place your hands in any comfortable posture.
- Hold for up to 1 minute.
- Then do the opposite side.

7. Heel-to-toe stroll

This workout strengthens your legs and improves balance.

- Stand with your heels pushed into a wall.
- Place your left foot in front of your right foot.
- Touch your left heel to your right toe.
- Then position your right foot in front of your right foot.
- Touch your right heel to your left toe.
- Continue for 20 steps.
- With a balancing board
- You'll need a balancing board for the following two workouts.
- Shop for balancing boards online.

8. Forward and backward tilt

- Stand with your feet on the outside borders of the balancing board.
- Shift your weight forward until the front of the board contacts the floor.
- Maintain this posture for a few seconds.
- Then move your weight backward until the back of the board meets the floor.
- Maintain this posture for a few seconds..

- Use deliberate, unhurried movements to keep tilting back and forth for 1 minute.

9. Single foot balancing

- Stand with your right foot positioned at the center of the board.
- Lift your left foot and raise your knee as high as possible.
- Hold this position for a duration of up to 30 seconds.
- Then do the opposite side.
- Repeat each side 2 to 3 times.
- With a walker

10. Marching

- Stand with both hands on your walker.
- Lift your left knee as far upward as possible.
- Lower it and then elevate your right knee.
- Switch sides after each repetition, completing a total of 20 repetitions.

11. Heel-toe rises

- Stand with both hands on your walker.
- Lift both heels off the ground and balance on the balls of your feet for 3 seconds.

- Then move the weight onto your heels and elevate your toes.
- Do 10 to 20 repetitions.

Day 18-20: Advanced Balance Techniques

Exercise 1: Single Limb Stance

It's better to start with a simple balancing exercise for seniors. Here's how you do this: stand behind a firm, solid chair (not one with wheels), and grab onto the back of it. Lift your right foot and balance on your left foot. Hold that posture for as long as you can, then swap your feet.

The objective should be to stand on one foot without hanging onto the chair and keep that stance for up to a minute.

Exercise 2: Walking Heel to Toe

You could read this and question, "How is walking an exercise to improve balance?" This exercise routine strengthens your legs, improving your stability for walking without the risk of falling.

Put your right foot in front of your left foot so that the heel of your right foot meets the top of the toes of your left foot. Shift your left foot forward, resting your weight on your heel while doing so. Then, move your weight to your toes. Repeat the step with your left foot. Walk in this direction for 20 steps.

Exercise 3: Rock the Boat

Stand with your feet apart, such that the space between them is the same width as your hips. Make sure both feet are planted into the ground firmly. Stand upright, with your head level. Then, transfer your weight to your right foot and carefully lift your left leg off the ground. Hold the posture for as long as possible (but no more than 30 seconds).

Slowly put your foot back onto the ground, then shift your weight to that foot. Slowly elevate your opposite leg. Start by practicing this exercise for balance five times per side, then work your way up to more repetitions.

Exercise 4: Clock Reach

You'll require a chair for this exercise.

Picture yourself positioned at the center of a clock. The number 12 is right in front of you and the number 6 is exactly behind you. Grip the chair using your left hand.

Lift your right leg and extend your right arm so it's pointing at the number 12. Next, point your arm toward the number three, and finally, aim it behind you toward the number 6. Move your arm from the three o'clock position to the twelve o'clock position. Look straightforward the whole time.

Repeat this exercise twice on each side.

Exercise 5: Back Leg Raises

This strength training routine for seniors makes your bottom and your lower back stronger.

Stand behind a chair. Slowly elevate your right leg straight back – don't bend your knees or point your toes. Hold that position for one second, then softly bring your leg back down. Repeat this 10 to 15 times per leg.

Exercise 6: Balancing on one leg while extending an arm

This balance exercise for seniors enhances your physical coordination.

Stand with your feet together and arms at your side close to a chair. Lift your left hand over your head. Then, carefully elevate your left foot off the floor. Hold that position for 10 seconds. Repeat the same operation on the right side.

Exercise 7: Side Leg Raise

You'll need a chair for this workout to enhance balance.

Stand behind the chair with your feet slightly apart. Lift your right leg gradually to the side. Keep your back straight, your toe facing front, and gaze straight ahead. Lower your right leg slowly. Perform this exercise on each leg 10 to 15 times.

Exercise 8: Balancing Wand

This balancing exercise for seniors may be completed while seated. You'll need a cane or any form of staff. A broomstick works nicely for this — simply remove the broom's head before you start.

Support the lower end of the stick so that it lies flat against your palm. The purpose of this workout is to maintain the stick straight for as long as possible. Change hands so that you focus on your balance abilities on both sides of your body.

Exercise 9: Wall Pushups

As long as you've got a wall, you may execute this strength training exercise for elders.

Stand about an arm's length away from a bare wall without paintings, decorations, windows, or doors. Lean forward slightly and place your palms flat against the wall, aligning them with your shoulders in both height and width. Keep your feet grounded as you gently pull your body towards the wall. Lean back gently until your arms are fully extended. Do twenty of these.

Exercise 10: Marching in Place

Marching is a fantastic balancing exercise for seniors. If you require support, perform this exercise facing a counter.

Standing straight, elevate your right knee as high as you can. Lower it, then elevate the left leg. Raise and lower your legs 20 times.

Exercise 11: Toe Lifts

This strength training routine for the elderly also improves balance. You'll need a chair or a counter.

Stand upright and place your arms in front of you. Raise yourself on your toes as high as you can go, then gently descend yourself. Avoid leaning excessively forward on the chair or counter. Lift and lower yourself 20 times.

Exercise 12: Shoulder Rolls

This is an easy workout for elders. You may perform it sitting or standing.

Rotate your shoulders gently upward towards the ceiling, then backward and downward. Next, do the same process, but roll them forward and then down.

Exercise 13: Hand and Finger Exercises

The following are exercises that enhance flexibility. You don't need to stand for these.

In the first exercise, assume there's a wall in front of you. Your fingers will climb the wall until they're over your head. While holding your arms over your head, wriggle your fingers for 10 seconds. Then, walk them back down.

During the second exercise, contact your hands while they're behind your back. Try this rephrased sentence: Extend your left hand towards you while keeping your right hand behind your back. Hold that posture for 10 seconds, then attempt with your other arm.

Exercise 14: Calf Stretches

These strength training routines for seniors can be performed sitting or standing.

To perform standing calf stretches, locate a clear wall. Stand facing the wall with your hands at eye level. Step your left leg behind your right, keeping your left heel on the ground and bending your right knee. Hold the stretch for 15 to 30 seconds. Repeat this sequence two to four times for each leg.

To stretch your calves while seated, you'll require a towel. Sit on the floor with your legs straight. Put the towel around the soles of your right foot and grip both ends. Pull the towel towards you while maintaining your knee straight and hold it for 15 to 30 seconds. Repeat the exercise two to four times each leg.

Day 21: Review and Reflect: Balancing Act

Congratulations on achieving Day 21 of your mindfulness journey! As you reflect on the last 21 days, take a minute to think about the concept of a balancing act.

Balancing Act:

Throughout the last 21 days, we've studied numerous mindfulness techniques to help you build balance in your daily life. This notion is vital for developing general well-being and minimizing stress. Balance is not simply about dividing your time and energy between different elements of your life, but also about achieving harmony inside yourself. It's about realizing that every moment has its own distinct needs and expectations and learning to adjust to those demands without feeling overwhelmed.

Reflective Questions:

1. What are some areas in your life where you struggle to find balance? (e.g., work-life balance, emotional balance, physical balance)

2. What are some tactics you've tried in the past to try to attain balance in those areas?

3. How have you observed your ability to balance has evolved over the past 21 days? Are there any new ideas or practices that have helped you reach more balance?

4. Are there any habits or routines that you've formed on your mindfulness journey that have led to increased balance in your life?

5. What are some issues you still experience in keeping balance, and how do you plan to handle them moving forward?

Mindfulness Exercise: Balancing Act Meditation

Find a comfortable sitting posture, close your eyes, and take a few deep breaths. Imagine yourself balancing on a tightrope, depicting the delicate balance between several parts of your life. Visualize each facet as a weight on each side of the tightrope. As you inhale, envision each weight increasing heavier, testing your equilibrium. As you exhale, envision each weight getting lighter, helping you to recover equilibrium.

Notice how you react to the fluctuations in weight. Do you feel worried or terrified when one side grows heavier? Do you feel more grounded when both sides are balanced? Take a few seconds to breathe into any tension or discomfort.

As you continue to breathe, envision yourself acquiring a sense of fluidity and flexibility. Envision yourself sliding easily over the tightrope, changing your weight with each breath. Remember that life is continuously changing, and equilibrium is not a set condition — it's a dynamic process.

Take one final deep breath, and when you're ready, carefully open your eyes.

Remember to be gentle and sympathetic with yourself as you continue to study the notion of the balancing act. It's a lifelong process, and little milestones can lead to great development over time.

Chapter 7

WEEK 4 - INTEGRATING STRENGTH, FLEXIBILITY, AND BALANCE

Day 22: Full-Body Engagement Sequence

Warm-Up (5 Minutes)

- Seated Cat-Cow Stretches: Begin by sitting comfortably with feet flat on the floor. Inhale, arch your back and elevate your chest (Cow Pose). Inhale, arch your back, and bring your chin towards your chest (Cat Pose). Repeat for 1 minute.
- Shoulder Rolls: Roll your shoulders forward for 1 minute, then backward for another minute to alleviate tension.

Main Sequence (15 Minutes)

- Seated Mountain Pose: Sit tall with hands on your knees, feet flat on the ground. Engage your core and take deep breaths for 1 minute.
- Seated Forward Bend: From Mountain Pose, hinge at your hips and reach for your toes. Hold for 3 deep breaths, then return to the starting position. Repeat 3 times.

- Chair Warrior II: Sit sideways on the chair, extend your right leg out, and bend your left knee to 90 degrees. Extend your arms parallel to the floor and glance over your right hand. Hold for 5 breaths, then swap sides.
- Seated Twist: Sit straight and place your right hand on the back of the chair and your left hand on your right knee. Inhale to stretch your spine, exhale to twist. Hold for 5 breaths, then swap sides.

Cool Down (5 Minutes)

- Seated Neck Stretches: Gently tilt your head to the right, bringing your right ear nearer your shoulder. Hold for 3 breaths, then swap sides. Repeat twice.
- Seated Relaxation: Sit back in your chair with your eyes closed. Focus on your breath, breathing, and expelling deeply for 2 minutes.

Day 23: Strength and Flexibility Sequence

Warm-Up (5 Minutes)

- Ankle Rotations: Lift one foot off the ground and spin your ankle clockwise for 30 seconds, then counterclockwise for another 30 seconds. Switch feet.
- Wrist Circles: Extend your arms and spin your wrists in both directions for 1 minute.

Main Sequence (15 Minutes)

- Seated Sun Salutations: Start with hands in prayer at your chest. Inhale, lift your arms overhead. Exhale, fold forward. Inhale, lift halfway up. Exhale, fold again. Inhale, raise back up with arms aloft. Exhale, return to prayer stance. Repeat 5 times.

- Chair Pigeon Pose: Sit with your feet flat on the floor. Place your right ankle on top of your left knee. Gently push down on your right knee to expand the hip. Hold for 5 breaths, then swap sides.

- Seated Leg Lifts: Sit tall with your hands on the chair for support. Lift one leg straight up and hold for 3 breaths, then lower. Repeat 5 times on each side.

- Chair Side Bend: Sit with feet flat and lift your right arm above. Bend to the left, maintaining your left hand on the chair for support. Hold for 5 breaths, then swap sides.

Cool Down (5 Minutes)

- Seated Forward Fold: Sit at the edge of your chair, legs outstretched. Hinge at your hips and reach toward your toes. Hold for 5 breaths, then gently raise back up.

- Deep Breathing: Sit comfortably with hands on your knees. Close your eyes and take slow, deep breaths for 2 minutes, concentrating on relaxation.

Day 24: Balance and Flow Sequence

Warm-Up (5 Minutes)

- Seated Marching: Sit tall and elevate one leg towards your chest, then drop. Alternate legs in a marching motion for 2 minutes.

- Finger Stretch: Extend your arms and extend your fingers wide. Hold for 5 seconds, and then create a fist. Repeat 10 times.

Main Sequence (15 Minutes)

- Seated Tree Pose: Sit with feet flat on the floor. Place your right foot on your left ankle or shin, avoiding the knee. Bring hands to prayer posture at your chest. Hold for 5 breaths, and then swap sides.

- Chair Warrior I: Sit sideways on the chair with your left leg bent at 90 degrees and your right leg stretched back. Raise your arms aloft and stare forward. Hold for 5 breaths, and then swap sides.

- Seated Eagle Pose: Cross your right thigh over your left and loop your right arm under your left, bringing palms together. Hold for 5 breaths, then swap sides.

- Seated Camel Pose: Sit at the edge of your chair, placing your hands on the backrest. Inhale, elevate your chest, and arch your back slightly. Hold for 3 breaths, then release. Repeat 3 times.

Cool Down (5 Minutes)

- Seated Spinal Twist: Sit tall and twist to the right, resting your left hand on your right knee and your right hand on the back of the chair. Hold for 5 breaths, then swap sides.
- Relaxation and Visualization: Sit comfortably, close your eyes, and take slow, deep breaths. Visualize a quiet environment and stay there for 2 minutes.

Tips for Success:

- Listen to your body: Only execute comfortable positions and change them as required.
- Stay well-hydrated by drinking water both before and after your practice.
- Consistency is key: Aim to practice regularly to optimize advantages.

By integrating these thorough sequences into your routine, you will boost your entire well-being, combining the advantages of strength, flexibility, and balance in a holistic practice.

Day 25-27: Full-Body Flow Practices

Day 25: Energizing Morning Flow

Warm-Up (5 minutes)

- Seated Cat-Cow Stretch: Begin with your hands on your knees. Inhale, arch your back and gaze up (Cow Pose).

Breathe out, arch your back, and gently lower your chin towards your chest (Cat Pose). Repeat for 5 breaths.

- Seated Side Stretch: Extend your left arm above and lean to the right. Hold for 3 breaths, then swap sides. Repeat twice on each side.

Main Flow (10 minutes)

1. Seated Mountain Pose: Maintain an upright posture with feet planted firmly on the floor and hands resting comfortably on your thighs. Inhale deeply, activating your core.

2. Seated Forward Bend: Exhale and hinge at your hips, bringing your hands towards the floor. Hold for 3 breaths.

3. Seated Warrior I: Place your left foot back and maintain your right knee bent. Raise your arms overhead. Hold for 5 breaths, then swap sides.

4. Seated Warrior II: Extend your arms out to the sides and glance over your right hand. Hold for 5 breaths, then swap sides.

5. Seated Twist: Place your right hand on the back of the chair and your left hand on your right knee. Twist slowly to the right. Hold for 5 breaths, then swap sides.

Cool Down (5 minutes)

- Seated Neck Stretches:Gently tilt your head to the right, bringing your right ear closer to your shoulder. Hold for 3 breaths, then swap sides.
- Seated Relaxation: Sit comfortably, close your eyes, and breathe deep, relaxing breaths for 2 minutes.

Day 26: Midday Revitalizing Flow

Warm-Up (5 minutes)

- Seated Shoulder Rolls: Roll your shoulders forward and backward for 10 reps each.
- Seated Chest Opener: Interlace your fingers behind your back and elevate your chest. Hold for 5 breaths.

Main Flow (10 minutes)

1. Seated Sun Salutation: Begin with hands in prayer position. Inhale, reach up. Exhale, forward bend. Inhale, lift halfway up. Exhale, and return to a forward bend. Inhale, raise back up, hands overhead. Exhale, return to prayer stance. Repeat 3 times.
2. Seated Chair Pose: Extend your arms forward and elevate your heels slightly off the floor. Hold for 5 breaths.
3. Seated Side Angle Pose: With feet wide apart, rest your right forearm on your right thigh and raise your left arm overhead. Hold for 5 breaths, then swap sides.

4. Seated Hamstring Stretch: Extend your right leg forward and grasp for your toes. Hold for 5 breaths, then swap sides.

5. Seated Eagle Arms: Cross your right arm across your left, bringing palms together. Lift elbows and hold for 5 breaths, then swap sides.

Cool Down (5 minutes)

- Seated Hip Opener: Place your right ankle on your left knee and bend forward gently. Hold for 5 breaths, then swap sides.

- Seated Meditation: Close your eyes, lay your hands on your knees, and focus on your breath for 2 minutes.

Day 27: Evening Relaxation Flow

Warm-Up (5 minutes)

- Seated Gentle Twist: Inhale, stretch your spine. Exhale, twist to the right. Hold for 3 breaths, then swap sides.

- Seated Wrist Stretches: Extend your right arm and softly pull back on your fingers with your left hand. Hold for 3 breaths, then swap sides.

Main Flow (10 minutes)

1. Seated Crescent Moon: Extend both arms aloft and lean to the right. Hold for 5 breaths, then swap sides.

2. Seated Pigeon Pose: Place your right ankle on your left knee and softly press down on your right knee. Hold for 5 breaths, then swap sides.

3. Seated Cow Face Arms: Raise your right arm above and bend your elbow, extending your hand down your back. Use your left hand to softly tug your right elbow.. Hold for 5 breaths, and then swap sides.

4. Seated Forward Fold with Extended Arms: Extend your arms forward and hinge at your hips to fold over your thighs. Hold for 5 breaths.

5. Seated Child's Pose: Slide your hands down your legs and fold forward, placing your forehead on your knees. Hold for 5 breaths.

Cool Down (5 minutes)

- Seated Ankle Rolls: Lift your right foot and spin your ankle in circles. Repeat 10 times in each direction, then swap sides.

- Seated Savasana: Sit comfortably with your hands on your lap, close your eyes, and focus on deep, slow breathing for 3 minutes.

Tips for Success:

- Listen to your body and alter positions as required.
- Use a solid chair without wheels to provide stability.

- Keep water available to remain hydrated.
- Practice mindfulness by concentrating on your breath and movements.

Day 28: Review and Reflect: Celebrating Your Achievements Congratulations! You've reached the final day of our 28-day chair yoga adventure. Today, we will take time to reflect on your progress, congratulate your victories, and set the scene for continuing success in your health journey. This is a day to appreciate your dedication, recognize your development, and feel proud of how far you've gone.

Reflecting on Your Journey

1. Revisit Your Goals:

- At the outset of this trip, you established particular goals for yourself. Take a few seconds to revisit these goals. Write them down if you haven't already.
- Reflect on the progress you've made. How have you progressed in terms of strength, flexibility, and balance? Have you seen any changes in your general well-being?

2. Measure Your Progress:

- Compare your present abilities to when you originally started. Use a notebook or a progress tracker to jot down particular improvements.

- Reflect on any physical improvements you've experienced, such as enhanced mobility, less discomfort, or improved posture.

3. Personal Milestones:

- Think about any personal milestones you've reached. These may include conquering a tough position, maintaining constancy in your practice, or experiencing a mental change towards a more positive approach.
- Celebrate these achievements, no matter how minor they may appear. Each step forward is a huge accomplishment.

Celebrating Your Achievements

1. Acknowledge Your Hard Work:

- Give yourself credit for the devotion and work you've put into this program. Completing a 28-day challenge is no minor achievement, and it's crucial to acknowledge and reward your hard work.
- Treat yourself to something unique. It might be a favorite meal, a peaceful hobby, or simply a tiny present that offers you delight.

2. Share Your Success:

- Consider sharing your triumphs with friends, family, or a supportive community. Sharing your success might inspire others and give you more motivation.

- If you feel comfortable, snap before-and-after images to visually chronicle your experience. These photographs might serve as a strong reminder of how far you've come.

3. Reflect on the Benefits:

- Take note of the advantages you've noticed beyond bodily improvements. How has this adventure influenced your mental and emotional well-being?
- Reflect on how chair yoga has changed your daily life. Do you feel more energized, less anxious, or more secure in your abilities?

Planning for the Future

1. Setting New Goals:

- Now that you've accomplished this challenge, think about what you want to achieve next. Setting fresh goals might help retain your drive and continue your success.
- Consider areas where you'd like to develop more or new parts of your well-being you'd like to focus on.

2. Maintaining Your Practice:

- Create a strategy to maintain your chair yoga practice. Consistency is crucial to long-term effects, so include yoga in your daily or weekly practice.
- Explore different positions and sequences to keep your practice fresh and entertaining. Challenge yourself to try more advanced maneuvers as your confidence improves.

3. Expanding Your Wellbeing Journey:

- Use the momentum from this challenge to investigate other facets of wellbeing. This might involve trying new types of exercise, optimizing your nutrition, or focusing on mental health techniques like meditation.
- Consider joining a neighborhood class or an online group to keep connected with individuals who share your wellness objectives.

Chapter 8

ADAPTING CHAIR YOGA TO YOUR NEEDS

How can I conduct a yoga class from the ground up?

The reality is, that a beginner yoga session might be one of the most demanding classes to train. They can also be one of the most fun and gratifying courses to instruct.

Here are the most helpful actions that I've acquired thus far for making a safe and pleasant newbie place.

1. Keep it simple

While it's vital to create the groundwork for a solid, healthy partnership, you don't want to provide beginners with so many recommendations and explanations that you confuse them. After all, our practical memory is restricted; when you're gaining a new talent, there's only so much that you can prepare at once.

When you're instructing beginners, it's a fantastic strategy to remain with the "basic form of the posture." This implies hardly safely directing them into the customary posture form (or a variant on that mold). From here, you might find it beneficial to add one or two further alignment tips. Alternatively, you might not.

Fix up the posture

This entails indicating which way the students should look, how long their stance should be, which help they should use and how they should handle them, where their hands and/or feet move, how to get into the posture, and whether they should start on an inhale or an exhale (if it indicates).

For instance, when introducing virabhadrasana II, you may say:

- Twist to face the long end of your mat, and step your feet wide isolated

- Turn your back foot in softly.

- Pivot on your forehead such that your front toes go toward the short end of the mat.

- On an exhale, rotate your front knee such that it gathers over your front heel.

- On an inhalation, drift your arms out to your sides to establish a "T" shape.

- On your next exhalation, turn your head to look at your front hand—only as much as feels acceptable for your neck.

- You're setting up the position here, directing on growing stable grounds, and constructing the shape itself by piling the bones on top of each other. That's it.

2. Create Transformations Uncomplicated

Turns may be tough. While leaping forward from the downward-facing dog, or springing through to a sitting is very typical in yoga courses, that doesn't imply they're comfortable! They may be extremely frustrating for plenty of learners. To foster confidence and minimize unneeded vexation, when you initially teach postures to new students, make your transitions easy.

Further, while you're moving to sitting it's appropriate to abandon the elaborate choreography and instead urge kids to "sit down" or "lie on your bellies." Keep things simple.

3: Go Easy On (and explain!)

Don't assume that pupils will instantly know what "energy lines," "employ Mula bandha," or "Anjali mudra" means. Use terminology that non-yogis will understand, and when you offer some new vocab, describe it! The same works for Asana styles.

The Greatest Method to Push Yourself?

Challenging yourself is a terrific way to improve personally and professionally. Here are some techniques to properly push yourself:

- Set Clear Goals: Define precise, measurable, attainable, relevant, and time-bound (SMART) goals that challenge you out of your comfort zone.

- Step Out of Your Comfort Zone: Challenge yourself to do new things or take on jobs that you find challenging. Growth typically comes when you push yourself beyond what you're used to.

- Continuous Learning: Always search for opportunities to gain new skills or enhance your knowledge in areas of interest. This might entail taking courses, reading books, or attending workshops.

- Seek Feedback: Feedback is vital for progress. Actively seek feedback from others to understand your strengths and places for growth.

- Embrace Failure: Failure is a normal component of progress. Don't be scared to fail, but instead, consider it as a chance to learn and better.

- **Stay Consistent:** Consistency is crucial to overcome problems. Break down your goals into smaller, doable activities and work on them frequently.

- **Surround Yourself with Supportive Individuals:** Surround yourself with individuals who challenge and encourage you. They may give encouragement, motivation, and useful insights.

- **Reflect on Your Progress:** Regularly reflect on your progress and alter your strategy as appropriate. Celebrate your accomplishments and learn from your setbacks.

- **Try New Experiences:** Stepping outside of your routine might help you find new hobbies and perspectives. Traveling, volunteering, or exploring new activities may all give fresh challenges.

- **Practice Mindfulness:** Being present in the moment will help you stay focused on your objectives and overcome challenges with a clear mind.

Remember, the key is to find a balance between establishing difficult objectives and ensuring they are practical and achievable. Challenging yourself should be a good experience that helps you grow and develop as an individual.

7 Ways to Personalize Your Yoga Practice

Here are seven ideas to help you customize your yoga practice and make your time on the mat a real representation of your intentions and individuality:

1. Set Your Intention: Your Unique Starting Point

Your yoga journey begins with intention. At the outset of each practice, create an aim that connects with your present needs and objectives. Whether your goal is to find relaxation, enhance flexibility, build strength, or foster a deeper connection with your inner self, this objective guides you.

2. Choose a Style That Fits You: Finding Your Yoga Path

Yoga provides a multitude of styles, each with its distinct attributes. Explore these numerous types, such as Hatha, Vinyasa, Ashtanga, or Kundalini, to find the one that most matches your interests and aspirations. Your choice of style will affect the adventure you take on each time you walk onto your mat.

3. Choose Poses That Suit Your Goals: Customizing Your Routine

The positions you pick are the building blocks of your practice. Select Asanas that directly connect to your objective. If you're wanting to develop balance, consider including positions like Tree or Warrior III. Seeking relaxation? Poses like Child's Pose or Happy Baby can be the perfect match.

4. Adapt for Your Body: Personalized Adjustments

Yoga is a personal experience, and your body has its unique demands and limits. Modify postures to adapt to your body's requirements. Props like blocks, belts, or bolsters maybe your friends in ensuring your practice is pleasant and accessible.

5. Craft Thoughtful Sequences: Developing a Balanced Routine

Your practice should flow effortlessly and fit with your aim. Craft sequences that begin with comfortable warm-up poses, flow into the selected asanas and close with a relaxing cool-down. This systematic strategy ensures your practice fits with your aims.

6. Breathe Mindfully: A Key Element

Your breath is the connection between your mind and body during your practice. Use it as a tool for focus, relaxation, and self-awareness. Experiment with various breathing methods, including Ujjayi, to enhance your practice.

7. Embrace Mindfulness: Present in the Moment

Immerse yourself entirely in your practice by letting go of distractions. Stay present, appreciate the feelings in your body, and be mindful of the thoughts in your head. Mindfulness brings depth and complexity to your particular yoga practice.

Chapter 9

THE ROLE OF NUTRITION

Eating for Energy: Understanding Nutritional Needs

Nutrition is the study of how food and beverages operate within the body. It is how our bodies take in micronutrients (vitamins and minerals) and/or macronutrients (carbohydrates, fats, and proteins) and use them to produce energy and develop. Nutrition is required for the basic processes of the human body.

Eating a Nutrient Diet

We have all heard the adage "You are what you eat", and there is truth to this. The meals we select to put into our bodies immediately affect how our bodies operate. The food we eat is broken down in our intestines and then used for energy to accomplish our physiological functions. Food is categorized into three types: proteins, carbs, and fats.

Proteins are building components that make biological systems operate and create muscle. Proteins are present in meat, fish, tofu, eggs, beans, yogurt, chickpeas, cheese, nuts & seeds.

Carbohydrates are sugars, starches, and fibers found in fruits, grains, dairy products like milk and ice cream, bread, cereals, juice, and legumes like beans, lentils, and peas, and in many meals they taste sweet/contain sugar. They provide us with fast energy by immediately boosting blood sugar.

Fats are utilized for fuel to make the body work; dietary fats maintain your skin and hair healthy and help you absorb certain key vitamins from meals. Good fats are unsaturated (especially mono-unsaturated) and are found in foods like olive oil, seafood, nuts, seeds, and avocados. In contrast, saturated fats are not as beneficial and should be ingested in lesser quantities. Eating too many saturated fats will elevate LDL ("bad") cholesterol, block your arteries, and increase your risk of heart attack and stroke. They are present in fried meals, butter, beef, certain cheeses, and dairy products.

What to Eat

When it comes to picking what to eat, keep things simple. Think about eating whole-natural foods that are minimally processed. Another way of stating it is to attempt to consume foods with the "fewest steps from farm to table"…meaning foods that aren't modified very much from when they were growing before you eat them. These foods will be the most nutrient-dense. These sorts of foods will leave you feeling full and content.

Processed foods should be taken rarely since they include significant quantities of salt, fat, and added sugars; these meals don't make you feel as content, leaving you hungry a short time later. They also have loads of fat, and calories, and may be pricey.

No items are off limits but remember to consume everything in moderation. Don't consume too much of any one food or kind of nutrient…meaning don't have most of your diet be just carbs or just fats or just protein. Your diet should be diverse with some of each vitamin.

Most of your diet should be packed with vegetables (especially green veggies), fruits, complete grains, and lean meats. According to the MyPlate Model (the national nutritional recommendation that replaced the "food pyramid"), vegetables and fruits should make up ½ (or 50%) of each meal and snack, whole grains ¼ (or 25%) of your plate, and protein ¼ (or 25%) of the plate.

Vegetables and fruits should be the bulk of what you consume since they help clear your arteries, give critical vitamins and minerals, and help your body work more effectively. They also assist minimize inflammation. Remember that fruits include squash, tomatoes, cucumbers, peppers, eggplant, pumpkins, and avocados. Be careful to restrict fruits with plenty of sugar including pineapple, watermelon, mangoes, grapes, and bananas.

Eating healthily does not need restriction. When selecting meals rich in nutrients, you'll find that you can consume more while feeling full faster and staying satisfied longer.

Boredom Eating

We are all guilty of boredom eating, so before you grab that handful of chips first try sipping a glass of water to check if you are hungry. After drinking water, go for a bunch of carrots instead of the chips. If you don't want the carrots, you are likely not hungry. Be more cautious while picking the sorts of food and when you are eating.

Eating While Standing

Avoid eating while standing. This can increase the quantity you consume, contribute to bloating, and lead to feeling hungry sooner.

Track What You Eat

An easy method to be more aware of the things you put into your body is to track your intake. You may accomplish this with a pen and paper or use one of the numerous free applications available. By merely recording your diet, you may find yourself making new choices. Mindful eating frequently leads to increased satisfaction in eating, eating healthier meals, and eating less.

Seek Nutritional Counseling

If you are still feeling overwhelmed about how to eat healthily, your primary care physician is ready to help and answer all your concerns. Don't feel scared to question your doctor about how to eat healthily. Remember that everybody is different and no one diet suits everyone.

Hydration Tips: Staying Properly Hydrated

Staying adequately hydrated is vital for sustaining overall health and well-being. Here are some easy methods to remain hydrated:

- Drink enough water: The easiest and most efficient strategy to keep hydrated is to drink enough water throughout the day. The basic advice is to drink at least eight 8-ounce glasses of water every day (approximately 2 liters). However, individual water demands may vary based on factors such as exercise level, climate, and general health.

- Carry a water bottle: Keep a reusable water bottle with you at all times, whether you're at work, school, or doing errands. Having water easily available will remind you to drink and make it more convenient to keep hydrated.

- Set reminders: If you regularly forget to drink water, put reminders on your phone or utilize hydration apps to alert you at regular intervals. These reminders might help you build a habit of drinking water throughout the day.

- Eat hydrating foods: Many fruits and vegetables have significant water content and can add to your overall hydration. Include items like melons, cucumbers, oranges, strawberries, and lettuce in your diet to enhance your water consumption.

- Monitor urine color: Keep an eye on the color of your urine to check your hydration levels. If your urine is pale yellow or clear, it suggests that you are well-hydrated. Dark yellow urine signals that you may need to consume more water.

- Drink before, during, and after physical activity: When you exercise or participate in physical activities that cause you to sweat, your body loses water. Make sure to drink water before, during, and after exercise to restore fluids and maintain hydrated.

- Limit caffeine and alcohol: Both caffeine and alcohol can have a diuretic effect, which means they increase urine output and may contribute to dehydration. If you consume these beverages, do so in moderation and balance them with proper water consumption.

- Flavor your water: If you find plain water uninteresting, add a slice of lemon, lime, cucumber, or a few berries to improve the taste. Infusing your water with natural tastes might make it more pleasurable and encourage you to drink more.

- Keep water visible: Place a glass or bottle of water within your line of sight, such as on your desk or kitchen counter. Seeing it will act as a visual reminder and remind you to drink water regularly.

- Be conscious of your hydration needs: Pay attention to your body's signs of thirst and respond swiftly by drinking water. Additionally, be careful of hot weather, excessive physical activity, or illness, since these factors may increase your requirement for water.

Remember, keeping sufficient hydration is an ongoing process, and it's crucial to make it a habit in your daily routine. By following these suggestions, you can guarantee you keep well hydrated and support your overall health.

What are some ideas for introducing more plant-based meals into one's diet?

Incorporating more plant-based foods into your diet can have several health and environmental benefits. Whether you're wanting to embrace a plant-based (vegan) diet or simply want to eat more plant-based meals, here are some recommendations to help you get started:

- Start Gradually: If you're new to plant-based eating, start by introducing one or two plant-based meals into your weekly routine. As you become more at ease, you can gradually add more plant-based meals to your diet.

- Experiment with veggies: Try different veggies, both cooked and raw, to discover new flavors and textures. Experiment with various cooking methods, such as roasting, sautéing, steaming, and grilling, to make veggies more appetizing.

- Discover Plant-Based Proteins: Integrate plant-derived protein options such as beans, lentils, tofu, tempeh, and seitan into your diet. These can serve as alternatives for animal proteins in many recipes.

- Whole Grains: Choose whole grains like brown rice, quinoa, bulgur, and oats over processed grains. They are richer in fiber and nutrients.

- Nuts and Seeds: Incorporate nuts such as almonds and walnuts, and seeds like chia seeds and flaxseeds, into your diet. They are good suppliers of healthy fats, protein, and different nutrients.

- Legumes: Beans, chickpeas, lentils, and peas are versatile foods that may be used in soups, stews, salads, and more. They contain significant amounts of protein and fiber.

- Plant-Based Dairy Substitutes: Consider transitioning to plant-based milk substitutes like almond, soy, oat, or coconut milk. You can also investigate plant-based cheese, yogurt, and butter replacements.

- Use Herbs and Spices: Experiment with herbs and spices to add flavor to your food. This can make plant-based meals more enticing and gratifying.

- Try Meat Alternatives: Explore plant-based meat substitutes including veggie burgers, plant-based sausages, and vegetarian crumbles. These products resemble the flavor and texture of meat.

- Plan Balanced Meals: Ensure that your plant-based meals are well-balanced and contain a range of foods to suit your nutritional needs. Include a supply of protein, lots of veggies, and nutritious carbohydrates.

- Learn New Recipes: Search for plant-based recipes online or in cookbooks to discover new foods and cooking techniques. There are innumerable imaginative and tasty plant-based meals available.

- Consume the Rainbow: Aim to consume a variety of colorful fruits and vegetables to increase your intake of vitamins, minerals, and antioxidants.

- Mindful Eating: Pay attention to portion amounts and practice mindful eating. This can help you prevent overeating and make your meals more pleasurable.

- Plan Ahead: Prepare plant-based snacks and meals in advance to make it simpler to keep to your nutritional objectives, especially when you're busy.

- Educate Yourself: Learn about the nutritional components of plant-based food to ensure you satisfy your dietary needs, especially for critical nutrients like vitamin B12, iron, and calcium. Consider meeting with a licensed dietician for tailored counsel.

Remember that plant-based eating may be flexible, and there's no one-size-fits-all strategy. Customize your plant-based diet to fit your interests and lifestyle while concentrating on balance and diversity. As you add more plant-based foods into your diet, you may discover that you enjoy the benefits of increased health and less environmental impact.

Chapter 10

DELICIOUS AND HEALTHY RECIPES

Energizing Breakfasts: Start Your Day Right

Let's face it - getting out of bed might often feel insurmountable. If you usually feel sleepy in the morning, keep in mind that the food you consume may make a great difference in providing you the energy and motivation to go through your day.

A balanced breakfast comprises protein, slowly digested carbs, and healthy fats, along with some fruit or vegetables. Here's why they're important:

Proteins These are utilized to create and repair tissue in your body, transport, and store nutrients, and give your body with energy.

Carbohydrates These are the major sources of energy for your body. Fiber is a form of carbohydrate that assists in digestion.

Fats These give energy and also assist your body to absorb some vitamins. Get enough monounsaturated or polyunsaturated fats, such as those found in almonds, avocados, and olive oil.

Adding the following meals or a mix of these products to your breakfast will give you the energy boost you need to get through your day.

1. Oatmeal

Your body converts food into energy. Foods heavy in carbs may be the simplest to convert into fuel.

But simple carbs, like sugar, tend to be consumed extremely rapidly. This implies they'll provide you with only a small burst of energy that'll run out rapidly.

For long-lasting energy, include a complex carbohydrate, such as oats and grains, in your meal.

Oatmeal without added sugar is one of your greatest alternatives. Oats are a complete grain cereal and a healthy source of carbs and fiber, along with some protein and fat.

Oats are also filled with vitamins and minerals, including:

- Manganese
- Phosphorus
- Magnesium
- Copper
- Iron
- Zinc

- Folate
- Vitamin B1

Due to their fiber content, oats will make you feel filled longer. In other words, oatmeal will deliver long-lasting fullness to carry you through your day.

Oatmeal may be consumed by cooking oats with water to produce porridge. You may then add a broad range of toppings or mix-ins, including:

- Fruit
- Protein powder
- Cocoa powder
- Nuts

Oats can also form the foundation of baked products like pancakes.

2. Almond butter

Almonds are an excellent source of:

- Fats
- Antioxidants
- Iron
- Calcium
- Vitamin E

Almonds also provide some protein.

Though heavy in fat, this is the type of fat you'd want for breakfast. Almond butter is strong in monounsaturated fat, a form of lipid-associated with a reduction in heart disease and better blood sugar control.

Two tablespoons of almond butter include around 3.3 grams of fiber and 6.7 grams of protein, which might mean you'll feel full for longer.

You may simply include almond butter into a smoothie or combine it with a hot dish of oats. When searching for almond butter, make sure to choose a brand that doesn't contain any added sugar, trans fats, or artificial additives.

Moderation is crucial when it comes to nut butter, as they're generally heavy in calories.

3. Eggs

Eggs are another power meal that is a terrific morning choice. One egg has 75 calories, along with 6 grams of protein and 5 grams of good fats.

They're a terrific alternative to create the basis of a nutritious breakfast. Eggs are also incredibly flexible. They may be prepared

into an omelet with veggies, scrambled, hard-boiled, soft-boiled –
the list goes on.

4. Greek yogurt

Greek yogurt is a good source of probiotics. These are living
bacteria that assist your gut stay healthy, so you won't have to
worry about feeling lethargic during the day owing to poor
digestion.

What's fantastic about Greek yogurt is how many different power
foods you can put on top. Berries, almonds, oats, granola, seeds,
honey, apples, papaya, mango, coconut, and over a dozen more
fruits may make breakfast a delightful and rewarding way to start
your day.

5. Papaya

Papayas are a fantastic complement to breakfast, in a smoothie
with coconut milk, for example, or added to yogurt. Or just chop it
up and eat it as a side dish.

This tropical delicacy is packed in fiber and antioxidants known as
carotenoids, as well as vitamins A and C.

Vitamin C can aid with the absorption of non-heme iron, which is
the form of iron present in plant-based meals. It can also assist in
maintaining your immune system.

However, since it's a water-soluble vitamin, it isn't easily stored in your body. So, you'll need to routinely eat foods rich in vitamin C to restore your storage.

6. Ground flaxseed

Ground flaxseed may take your breakfast to the next level. Flax is abundant in soluble fiber, which might help delay digestion and reduce your blood sugar. If you tend to nibble between meals, adding flaxseed to your breakfast may aid in fending off hunger sensations.

Sprinkle a couple of tablespoons of ground flaxseed onto your porridge or yogurt, or try adding it to a smoothie or baked goods. You may prepare a flax "tea" by combining it with hot water, lemon juice, honey, and spices.

7. Berries

Blueberries, strawberries, raspberries, and blackberries are generally considered superfoods. They're abundant in antioxidants, fiber, and vitamin C.

Though they may taste sweet, berries are often low in calories, so you don't have to stint on them. Even folks on a low-carb and ketogenic diet can eat berries in moderation.

Berries may be readily included in smoothies prepared with almond, oat, dairy, or coconut milk, or can be added to oatmeal or yogurt. They also make a terrific mid-morning snack.

8. Chia seeds

Chia seeds are a significant source of fiber. The kind of fiber in chia seeds is a viscous fiber, which means it absorbs water. As the meal goes through your digestive tract, it will grow in volume.

Adding only a teaspoon or two of chia seeds to your breakfast might mean feeling full for much longer.

You may also experiment with a range of various chia seed puddings produced by mixing chia seeds with milk. As the chia seeds absorb the milk and swell, it creates a pudding-like consistency.

Here's a recipe for a protein-packed chia seed pudding that's guaranteed to make your day better:

- 3 tbsp. chia seeds
- 2 tbsp. protein powder
- 3/4 cup unsweetened almond milk (or milk of choice)
- 1 tbsp. cocoa powder
- 1/2 tbsp. maple syrup (or similar amount of sweetener of choice)

- Pinch of salt

In a bowl, combine all ingredients. Cover and chill in the refrigerator for a minimum of 1 hour. Before consuming, you may top with berries or coconut flakes or mix in 1 tbsp. almond butter for an additional energy boost.

9. Avocado

There's a solid reason why avocado toast became the current morning sensation. Avocados are a fruit providing a broad array of nutrients, including healthy fats, vitamins, and minerals.

Avocados contain:

- Vitamin K
- Folate
- Vitamin c
- Potassium
- B vitamins
- Vitamin e

Avocado may be put atop an omelet or crushed into whole-grain bread. You may also add it to a smoothie to give the drink a creamy smoothness.

10. Coconut

Coconuts supply largely fat, but they also provide numerous vital minerals and modest levels of B vitamins.

The high fiber content of coconut flesh can also aid delay digestion and managing blood sugar levels.

Flaked or shaved coconut provides a delightful taste to sweet breakfast meals. Try it on top of yogurt, cereal, or cottage cheese together with other fruits, such as mangoes or berries.

The takeaway

Adding any of these things to your breakfast may give you the extra push you need to make it through a hectic day.

Many of these meals provide a healthy dosage of fiber to slow down digestion and keep you full. The vitamins and antioxidants mixed with protein and healthy fats are likely to help you feel refreshed as you go about your day.

To get the most out of your morning meal, aim for a breakfast that includes protein combined with slowly digested carbs, healthy fats, and fruits or vegetables.

Chapter 11

LIGHT AND NUTRITIOUS LUNCHES: KEEP YOUR ENERGY UP

Story on healthy lunch choices:

Hey there! Let's speak about lunch, that noon meal that powers us through the remainder of the day. Choosing the correct meals for lunch is crucial to keeping our energy up and our bodies feeling well.

When it comes to a nutritious lunch, contemplate balance. You want a balance of nutrients that'll keep you satiated and focused until supper. Here are some fantastic ideas to consider:

1. Veggies, Veggies, Veggies!

Load up on colorful foods like spinach, carrots, bell peppers, and cucumbers. They're rich in vitamins, minerals, and fiber that keep you full and your body happy. You may toss them in a salad, put them in a wrap, or enjoy them as a side dish.

2. Lean Protein Power

Proteins are the building blocks of a nutritious meal. Go for lean alternatives like grilled chicken, turkey, tofu, beans, or fish. They offer you the energy you need and help your muscles stay strong.

3. Smart Carbs

Choose nutritious grains like brown rice, quinoa, or whole-grain bread for your carb fix. These provide you with enduring energy and won't leave you crashing an hour later. They are also rich in fiber, which aids digestion.

4. Healthy Fats

Yes, fats may be healthy! Avocado, almonds, seeds, and olive oil are fantastic sources of healthful fats. They keep your heart happy and help you feel full longer.

5. Hydration Station

Don't forget to drink water! Sometimes our bodies confuse thirst with hunger, so staying hydrated might help suppress those noon cravings.

Lunch Ideas to Try:

- Veggie Stir-fry: Load it up with colorful veggies, healthy protein, and a side of brown rice.
- Salad Power: Mix your favorite greens with some protein (chicken, tofu, or chickpeas), toss in nuts, seeds, and a drizzle of olive oil for a filling dinner.
- Wrap It Up: Use whole-grain wraps loaded with turkey, hummus, vegetables, and a sprinkling of cheese.

Quick Tips:

- Prep Ahead: Spend a little time planning your lunches for the week. It saves time and protects you from grabbing anything harmful.
- Portion Control: Monitor portion sizes. Eating too much, even nutritious food, can contribute to undesirable weight gain.

Remember, it's not about tight diets or restricting yourself. It's about making good decisions that nurture your body. Finding what works for you and your taste buds is crucial. And if you slip up now and again, don't sweat it! It's all about balance.

So, next time you're thinking about lunch, strive for that bright platter full of goodies. Your body will thank you for it!

Stay healthy and happy eating!

Disclaimer:

Before making any big adjustments to your diet or picking particular meals for your lunch or supper, it's crucial to talk with your healthcare professional, nutritionist, or a competent health coach. Everyone's body is different, and particular health issues or allergies could impact what's best for you.

The information supplied in this material is for general knowledge purposes only. It's not meant to substitute expert medical advice or specific dietary recommendations. Each person's nutritional demands differ, and what works well for one individual may not be good for another.

Always prioritize your health and well-being by getting tailored assistance from a healthcare expert or a qualified health coach before beginning on any new diet or meal plan.

Chapter 12

STAY EDUCATED, STAY HEALTHY!

Wholesome Dinners: End Your Day on a Healthy Note

Introduction

The Importance of a Balanced Dinner

Dinner is not merely the final meal of the day; it plays a significant part in preserving overall health and well-being. A balanced meal delivers the necessary nutrients to assist your body recover from the day's activities, encourages sound sleep, and sets the tone for the next day. For seniors, especially those engaged in regular chair yoga, it's crucial to focus on diets that promote muscle healing, increase flexibility, and maintain energy levels.

Key Components of a Wholesome Dinner

1. Lean Proteins: Essential for muscle repair and development. Sources include poultry such as chicken and turkey, seafood like fish, as well as plant-based options such as beans, lentils, and tofu.

2. Whole Grains: Provide steady energy and fiber. Examples include brown rice, quinoa, whole wheat pasta, and barley.

3. Colorful Vegetables: Packed with vitamins, minerals, and antioxidants. Aim for a diversity of hues to guarantee a wide spectrum of nutrients.

4. Healthy Fats: Support heart health and brain function. Include sources include olive oil, avocado, almonds, and seeds.

5. Hydration: Adequate fluids are vital, so consider soups or broths as part of your diet.

Sample Wholesome Dinner Recipes

1. Pan-Seared Salmon with Quinoa and Steamed Veggies

Ingredients

- 4 ounce salmon fillet
- 1 cup cooked quinoa
- 1 cup mixed veggies (broccoli, carrots, bell peppers)
- 1 tbsp olive oil
- Lemon juice, salt, and pepper to taste

Instructions:

1. Preheat the grill to medium-high heat.

2. Brush the salmon with olive oil and season with lemon juice, salt, and pepper.

3. Grill the salmon for 4-6 minutes on each side until well done.

4. Steam the veggies until tender.

5. Serve the grilled salmon over a bed of quinoa with a side of steamed veggies.

2. Chicken and Vegetable Stir-Fry

Ingredients:

- 1 chicken breast, thinly sliced
- 2 cups mixed veggies (snow peas, bell peppers, onions, mushrooms)
- 1 tsp. low-sodium soy sauce
- 1 tsp. olive oil
- 1 clove garlic, minced
- 1 tsp. ginger, grated
- 1 cup brown rice, cooked

Instructions:

- Heat olive oil in a large pan over medium heat.
- Cook the ginger and garlic until they release their aroma.
- Cook the chicken pieces until they are browned and done.

- Coat the veggies with soy sauce and stir-fry them until they are crisp-tender.
- Pile cooked brown rice on top of the stir-fry.

3. Lentil and Vegetable Stew

Ingredients:

- 1 cup green or brown lentils, washed
- 1 carrot, diced
- Diced celery, one stalk
- 1 onion, chopped
- 2 cups spinach leaves
- 4 cups vegetable broth
- 1 tsp. olive oil
- 1 tsp. cumin
- Salt and pepper to taste

Instructions:

1. Heat olive oil in a big saucepan over medium heat.
2. Add onion, carrot, and celery, sautéing until softened.
3. Add lentils, cumin, salt, and pepper, stirring to mix.
4. Pour in vegetable broth, bringing to a boil.
5. Reduce heat and simmer for 25-30 minutes until lentils are cooked.
6. Stir in spinach leaves and simmer until wilted.

7. Serve hot with a serving of whole-grain toast.

Tips for Creating Wholesome Dinners

- Plan Ahead: Prepare ingredients in advance to make cooking quicker and easier.
- Batch Cooking: Make bigger amounts and store leftovers for future meals.
- Variety: Rotate various proteins, grains, and veggies to make meals interesting and healthily balanced.
- Mindful Eating: Focus on eating deliberately and savoring each mouthful, which can assist digestion and boost enjoyment.
- Smart Snacking: Healthy Options Between Meals

There are many healthful snack alternatives you may enjoy between meals. Here are some ideas:

Fresh Fruit: Fruits including apples, bananas, cherries, oranges, and grapes are terrific choices. They are naturally delicious, and rich in vitamins, minerals, and fiber.

Vegetable Sticks: Carrot sticks, cucumber slices, bell pepper strips, and cherry tomatoes are low in calories and high in nutrients. They are wonderful with hummus or a yogurt-based dip.

Nuts and Seeds: Almonds, walnuts, pistachios, pumpkin seeds, and sunflower seeds are nutritious snacks filled with healthy fats, protein, and fiber. Just be aware of portion amounts as they are calorie-dense.

Greek Yogurt: Greek yogurt is a wonderful source of protein and calcium. You may add fruits, nuts, or a drizzle of honey for added taste.

Whole Grain Crackers with Cheese: Opt for whole grain crackers combined with a modest quantity of cheese for a delicious and balanced snack.

Hard-Boiled Eggs: Hard-boiled eggs are high in protein and can keep you feeling full for longer.

Popcorn: Air-popped popcorn is a whole-grain snack that can be a rich source of fiber. Just be mindful of additional butter or salt.

Smoothies: Blend fruits, veggies, yogurt, and a beverage of your choosing (such as water or almond milk) for a nutrient-packed snack.

Homemade Energy Balls: Make your energy balls using materials like oats, almonds, seeds, dried fruit, and nut butter. They are easy to prepare and may be kept for a few days.

Edamame: Edamame (young soybeans) are a fantastic source of plant-based protein and may be consumed steamed or roasted with a sprinkling of salt.

Remember to pick snacks that are balanced, containing protein, healthy fats, and fiber to help keep you satiated until your next meal. Also, be cautious of meal amounts to avoid overeating.

Chapter 13

CONNECTING MIND AND BODY

The Importance of Meditation: Enhancing Your Practice

Starting your day with yoga and meditation may provide various benefits not only in your health but also in your job life.

In our world full with technologies, mindful meditation might assist you improve your professional abilities. By integrating meditation in daily life, you may focus better. You will experience big improvements in work-life with greater productivity.

As a medical practitioner, I can state when performed frequently, meditation results in an increased number of activated genes that assist to battle serious health disorders. It is an excellent pharmaceutical therapy with no negative effects. By lowering the generation of free radicals, it slows down the aging process.

Meditation calms you by greatly lowering stress. By clearing your mind, it trains you to focus on one item at a time.

Whether you are seeking for health advantages or mental power, meditation is the solution with no ill effects.

One of the biggest misunderstandings regarding meditation is that it should cease the cognitive process. The basic purpose of meditation is not to halt your thoughts but to create awareness of your inner self. Meditation is embracing all your ideas and letting them go. It is not about turning off your thoughts, rather, comprehending them better. Meditation is training your mind to build a good outlook.

Some additional fallacies include, you should sit cross-legged while meditation, your mind should be calm, and it takes years to understand meditation.

The most fundamental belief of meditation is being nonjudgmental about oneself. When you practice meditation, there is no right method or wrong way. You can sit in a comfortable position, and if ideas invade your head, you should bring your attention back to the current moment. With some regularity, it will get simpler.

Meditation boosts your quality of life, giving greater concentration and optimism.

Why is it useful to meditate?

Meditation is like Multivitamins for your Brain. Good to take it every day.

It enlightens your body and relieves your mind and resulting in Happy soul.

1. Helps in reducing Depression, Anxiety
2. High blood pressure persons are highly advantageous
3. Reduces Stress 4. Helps in attaining emotional well-being
4. Enhances self-esteem and self -acceptance
5. Lessens Fear and loneliness
6. Increases mental strength and focus 8. Better decision making and issue solving
1. 9. Helps in creating optimistic mindset
2. 10. Better social relationships
3. 11. Better cognitive thinking and creative thinking
4. 12. Better decision making and issue solving
5. 13. Helps in avoiding arguments
6. 14. Helps in acquiring Better mood
7. 15. Encourages a healthy lifestyle
8. 16. Slows aging

Guided Relaxation Techniques: Finding Inner Peace

Inner serenity isn't something you "find", it's something you ARE. It merely looks to be not present, but that's only because attention has been conditioned to search "out there" for it. Striving to obtain any particular object or scenario or to relieve some imagined load keeps focus concentrated outwards, and when you do that inner peace will be forgotten. That drive has been conditioned into human thought, and it's that compulsion that has to be weakened by being comfortable with this current moment. So, without straining in any manner to locate anything simply be present to this particular moment as it is, without attempting to alter anything about it. Make no attempt to criticize, modify, label or characterize anything seen, heard, felt, touched, or tasted - simply be entirely and unconditionally open to it all.

Becoming totally present to what is, just as it is, without agenda to grasp onto or reject anything, brings forth the inner serenity that is already present. This instant is where existence occurs, where truth exists and remaining in this moment mindfully shows the footprint of what you are, serenity itself.

Because inner peace isn't something you discover (because you are already it) it can't be lost. What can be discovered may be lost. Logically, what you are must be completely present continually, therefore it can never be lost. However, it can be neglected. When inner serenity feels absent check where attention has gone. Typically it will move to mental activity; ideas about the future with accompanying fears or recollections of the past with related regrets or affection of previous experiences. Or focus will move on physical feelings that are typically painful. Wherever attention travels it will begin mental activity around whatever experience is developing, and getting caught up in that mental stream of ideas will eclipse the inner tranquility of your actual nature.

Now, I don't intend to imply that ideas should be considered as some type of adversary or should be suppressed. It's only that the "noisiness" of thinking shuts out the stillness of the ever present inner serenity of what you are, consciousness.

When attention is no longer drawn in an external direction and is allowed to merely settle down into its source, real nature/consciousness, inner calm steps forth effortlessly. And along with that inner serenity comes an inner quiet and silence. As you become more and more attentive to this, abidance begins to take root, and tranquility is felt more and more throughout all action. Over time you will sense inner serenity even while mind stream is busy, even in the middle of physical activity or emotional swings.

Appendix

QUICK REFERENCE MATERIALS

Recipe Index: Quick Access to Your Favorite Meals

Make Your Recipe Book Template

Do you find yourself continuously searching through your kitchen cabinets, attempting to discover that one dish you love? Or do you have a collection of recipes strewn throughout multiple cookbooks, online, and printouts, making it a Herculean chore to organize and discover them when you need them the most? If you answered yes to any of these questions, it's time to Make Your Recipe Book Template. In this blog article, we'll lead you through the process, step by step, so you may finally bring order to your culinary chaos.

The Recipe for Recipe Organization

Imagine having all your favorite recipes neatly arranged in one location, accessible at your fingertips anytime you're ready to cook up a wonderful supper. That's the joy of developing your recipe book template. It's not only about keeping your recipes in order; it's about changing your culinary experience into a smooth, delightful trip.

Why Create Your Recipe Book Template?

Before we go into the nitty-gritty of building your template, let's explore why it's worth the work.

Recipe Personalization

When you construct your recipe book template, you have the opportunity to modify it according to your tastes. You may customize the layout, fonts, and colors that connect with your culinary style.

Easy Accessibility

With a personalized recipe book, you won't have to browse through a hodgepodge of recipes again. Everything you need will be exactly where you want it, making your cooking sessions more efficient and pleasurable.

Ingredients for Your Recipe Book

Now that you're persuaded of the benefits, let's gather the elements you'll need to build your recipe book template.

Materials

To get started, you'll need some basic materials:

- A strong binder or notebook
- Sheet protectors or transparent plastic sleeves
- Printer and paper
- Pens, markers, or colored pencils for ornamentation
- Sections and Categories

Consider how you would like to arrange your recipes. Common sections include:

- Appetizers Main Courses
- Desserts Beverages
- Special Occasions
- Recipe Layout

Consider the arrangement of your recipes. Here are some components to include:

- Recipe title Ingredients list
- Cooking directions
- Prep time and cook time
- Servings
- Notes or personal tips
- The Creative Process

Now, let's get creative! This is where you can incorporate your individuality into your recipe book template.

Cover Design

Design a beautiful cover for your recipe book. You may embellish it with drawings, utilize family photographs, or apply your artistic abilities to make it truly yours.

Handwritten Touch

Consider writing out your favorite recipes in your handwriting. This gives a personal touch that no written recipe can match.

Recipe Notes

Leave an area for personal notes and tales. Did you adapt a recipe and make it your own? Share your cooking exploits with the directions.

Organizing Your Recipes

Once you've gathered your components and added a creative twist, it's time to organize your recipes.

Sorting

Sort your recipes into their relevant categories. This will make it much easier to find what you're searching for when the culinary bug hits.

Alphabetical or Chronological

Decide whether you want to order your recipes alphabetically or chronologically. Alphabetical is wonderful for rapid reference, while chronological may tell a tale of your culinary experience.

Index or Table of Contents

Include an index or table of contents at the beginning of your recipe book. This will operate as your recipe GPS, bringing you to the proper page.

Digital Recipe Templates

In this digital age, you may also design a virtual recipe book template. There are different apps and tools available for this purpose.

Online Platforms

Explore online platforms and apps that allow you to save and organize your recipes digitally. You may access them from your computer, tablet, or smartphone.

Customizable Templates

Many recipe applications feature adjustable templates, so you can still add your touch even in the digital environment.

Conclusion

Producing your recipe book template is not only about arranging recipes; it's about producing a culinary masterpiece that represents your style and personality. Whether you like the tactile feel of a physical book or the ease of a digital version, the option is yours.

So, gather your recipes, unleash your imagination, and go on this joyful voyage of building your very own recipe book template. Your cooking escapades will never be the same again. Happy cooking!

Incorporating your recipes into a personalized template is like creating a symphony of flavors and memories. It's like having a secret treasure vault of gastronomic pleasures waiting to be unearthed. So, why wait? Start today, and let the recipe book-making fun begin!

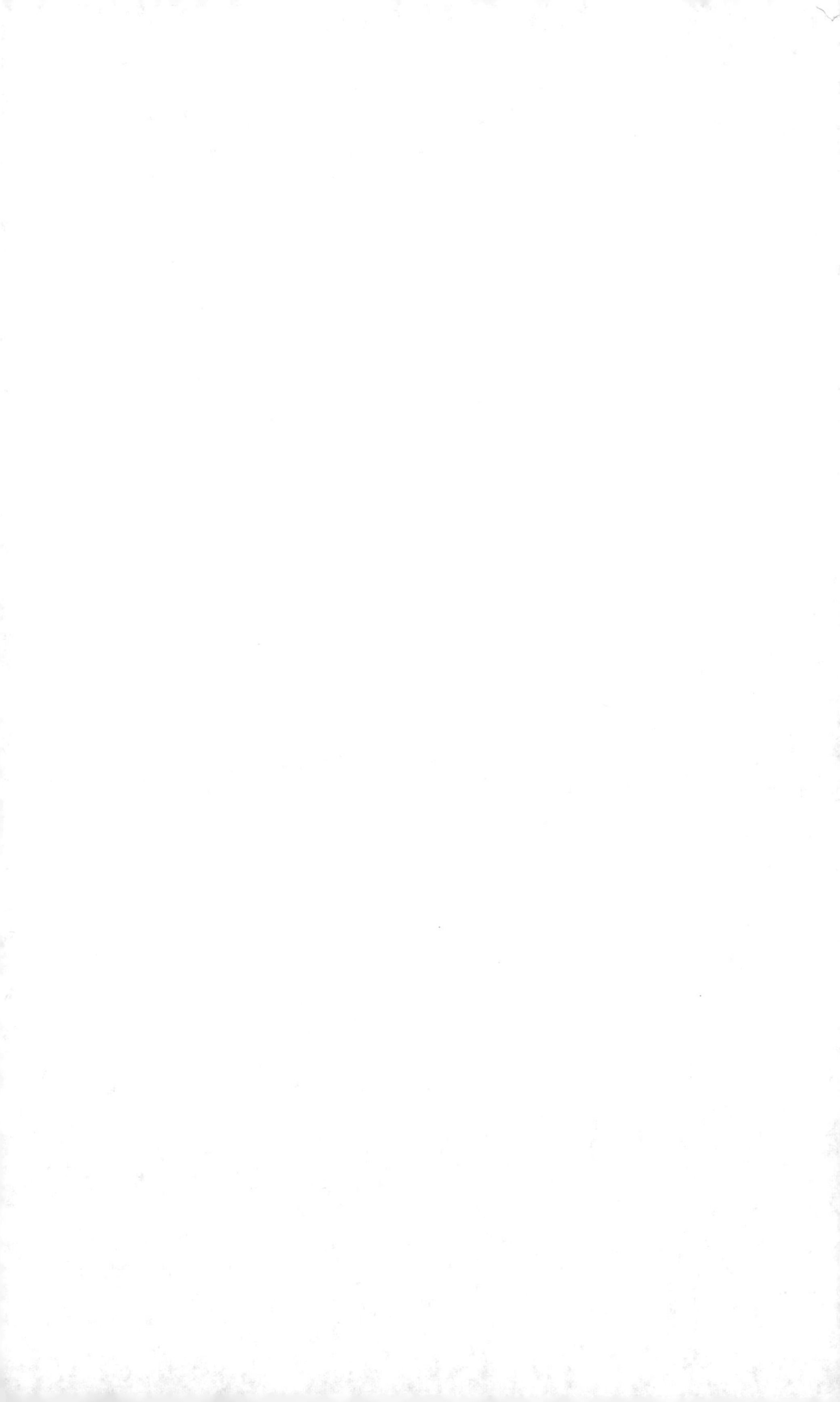